Fertility Endoscopy
Indications and Techniques

Akmal El-Mazny

Copyright © 2018 Akmal El-Mazny

All rights reserved.

CreateSpace, Charleston SC, USA

ISBN-13: 978-1986822992
ISBN-10: 1986822990

CONTENTS

	PAGE
INTRODUCTION	1

LAPAROSCOPY

– EVOLUTION OF LAPAROSCOPY	2
– INDICATIONS OF LAPAROSCOPY	4
– EQUIPMENT OF LAPAROSCOPY	12
– RELEVANT ANATOMY	21
– TECHNIQUE OF LAPAROSCOPY	23
– COMPLICATIONS OF LAPAROSCOPY	34
– CONTRAINDICATIONS OF LAPAROSCOPY	42
– EFFICACY OF LAPAROSCOPY	45

HYSTEROSCOPY

– EVOLUTION OF HYSTEROSCOPY	47
– INDICATIONS OF HYSTEROSCOPY	49
– EQUIPMENT OF HYSTEROSCOPY	57
– RELEVANT ANATOMY	67
– TECHNIQUE OF HYSTEROSCOPY	68
– COMPLICATIONS OF HYSTEROSCOPY	74
– CONTRAINDICATIONS OF HYSTEROSCOPY	78
– EFFICACY OF HYSTEROSCOPY	79

REFERENCES	80

INTRODUCTION

In gynecology, endoscopes are used most often to diagnose and treat conditions by direct visualization of the peritoneal cavity (laparoscopy) or the inside of the uterus through a transcervical approach (hysteroscopy).

For the evaluation of fertility, ovarian, tubal and uterine structures may be visualized using a variety of techniques including laparoscopy and hysteroscopy.

Laparoscopy is indicated mainly for the investigation of infertility, as well as the diagnosis and treatment of endometriosis and adhesions.

Hysteroscopy is considered the gold standard technique for the diagnosis and treatment of many intrauterine conditions.

It is essential that the surgeon fully understands all aspects of the use of the endoscopic equipment, and should be aware of the potential risks of the procedure.

Hopefully this book will enhance your knowledge of gynecological endoscopies along with their appropriate indications and use in infertility, and you will be able to apply this to your professional practice.

LAPAROSCOPY

EVOLUTION OF LAPAROSCOPY

The human dream was to see the "interior of the body".

During the last 35 years, gynecologic laparoscopy has evolved from a limited surgical procedure used only for diagnosis and tubal ligations to a major surgical tool used to treat a multitude of gynecologic indications.

Laparoscopy was first performed in dogs in the early 1900s by Dr. Georg Kelling, a German surgeon, who called his procedure "koelioskopie".

Dr. Hans Christian Jacobaeus, a Swedish surgeon, was the first to publish a description of "laparothorakoskopie" in humans in 1910.

Shortly thereafter, Dr. Bertram M. Bernheim of the Johns Hopkins Hospital, reported a series of the first human laparoscopy performed in the United States, which he called "organoscopy".

Throughout the 1920s and 1930s, advocates of the procedure continued to develop improved laparoscopic equipment.

During this period, Dr. Janos Veress, a Hungarian internist, developed a spring-loaded needle with an inner stylet that automatically converted the sharp cutting edge to a rounded end.

The Veress needle continues to be used today to create a pneumoperitoneum.

In 1924, Zollikofer used carbon dioxide (CO_2) instead of air to create a pneumoperitoneum.

A major step forward was the development of a safer laparoscopic cold lighting system in the 1950s.

LAPAROSCOPY: Evolution

Dr. Raoul Palmer, a French gynecologist who specialized in infertility, was an early pioneer in the development of laparoscopy in the mid 20th century.

In addition to advocating monitoring of intra-abdominal pressure, he expanded the therapeutic use of laparoscopy.

In 1961, Dr. Palmer described the first laparoscopic retrieval of oocytes, and in 1974 he described the point 3 cm below the last rib in the left mid-clavicular line.

Palmer's point is often used today for left upper quadrant laparoscopic entry.

Dr. Kurt Semm, a German gynecologist who specialized in infertility, was the most influential early advocate of modern operative laparoscopy.

In the 1960s and 1970s, Dr. Semm invented the automatic insufflator, and hundreds of laparoscopic instruments.

He was one of the first proponents of video monitoring for laparoscopy.

He developed many laparoscopic surgical techniques.

In recent years, 3 innovations that have been introduced or reintroduced to the field of endoscopy:

– Robotic surgery.

– Natural Orifice Transluminal Endoscopic Surgery (NOTES).

– Single Incision Laparoscopic Surgery (SILS).

Currently, laparoscopy is one of the most common surgical procedures performed by gynecologists.

INDICATIONS OF LAPAROSCOPY

Laparoscopy may be diagnostic or operative.

Diagnostic laparoscopy is indicated mainly for investigation of subfertility and pelvic pain.

It is also the standard method for the diagnosis of endometriosis and adhesions, as no other imaging technique provides the same degree of sensitivity and specificity.

Other indications include: ectopic pregnancy, PID (including TB), adnexal torsion, congenital pelvic abnormality, abnormal pelvic scan, and staging for ovarian malignancy.

Operative laparoscopy enables a physician to do complex, delicate procedures through small incisions, thus decreasing the patient's discomfort, morbidity, expense and duration of convalescence.

There are both diagnostic and therapeutic indications for laparoscopy in infertile women:

– Tubal patency and mobility can be directly observed via the laparoscope.

– Laparoscopy is able to confirm or rule out intrinsic pelvic disorders, such as endometriosis or chronic PID.

– Laparoscopic treatment of infertility includes operations used to reconstruct the normal anatomic relationships altered by an inflammatory process such as fimbrioplasty, adhesiolysis, and salpingostomy for distal obstruction.

Laparoscopic operations for the treatment of mechanical infertility are probably equally effective to similar procedures performed by laparotomy.

In patients with extensive adhesions, however, the effectiveness of all procedures is limited. IVF is necessary in these situations.

Hydrosalpinges

A hydrosalpinx, or fluid-filled tube, occurs after an inflammatory process damages the serosa and mucosa of the fallopian tube, creating an occlusion in the distal part of the tube.

As a result, normal and pathologic secretions may accumulate in the tube.

The frequency of hydrosalpinges in distal tubal disease is approximately 10% to 30%.

There has been considerable controversy as to the best and most appropriate surgical intervention for hydrosalpinges.

Less invasive procedures like needle aspiration of hydrosalpinx fluid, salpingostomy, fimbriolysis, and proximal tubal occlusion have been proposed.

Tubo-Ovarian Abscess (TOA)

Tubo-ovarian abscess is part of a spectrum of inflammatory disorders of the upper female genital tract comprising PID that includes any combination of endometritis, salpingitis, pelvic peritonitis, and TOA.

The primary aim of management of TOA is to be as conservative as possible, because most women with TOA are of reproductive age.

Patients who do not improve under antibiotic therapy usually require hospitalization, additional diagnostic tests, and surgical intervention.

Laparoscopic procedures in women with TOA usually comprise draining and irrigation of the abscess or complete removal of the inflamed tube or adnexa, in addition to pelvic irrigation and lysis of adhesions.

Lysis of Adhesions

Adhesions may form following infection, such as a ruptured appendix or PID, endometriosis, or previous surgery.

Adhesions may contribute to infertility or chronic pelvic pain.

Any of the electrosurgical instruments may be used for blunt or sharp dissection and coagulation.

Aquadissection may aid in the development of planes prior to lysing.

Minimal use of electrocautery and good hemostasis can help in reducing the chance of adhesions reformation.

Unfortunately, adhesiolysis is often ineffective in curing chronic pelvic pain and improving future fertility.

The chances of pregnancy after lysis of adhesions is relatively low for most patients, and this type of surgery has been largely followed by IVF.

Endometriosis

Endometriosis is classically defined as the presence of uterine endometrial glands and stroma outside the normal location-mainly on the pelvic peritoneum, but also on the ovaries, and in the rectovaginal septum, and more rarely in the pericardium, pleura, and even the brain.

Endometriosis is commonly found in women of reproductive age.

Endometriosis may be either asymptomatic or associated with minor symptoms and lesions that are sometimes self-limiting.

Sometimes it may be associated with severe symptoms and major pathologic lesions involving the vital structures of the pelvis.

Patients with endometriosis may suffer from dysmenorrhea, dyspareunia, chronic pelvic pain, and/or subfertility, which may result in reduced quality of life, psychologic morbidity, and work absenteeism.

Level of therapeutic intervention depends on age of the patient, extent of the disease, severity of the symptoms, and desire for fertility.

Laparoscopic diagnosis and excision of all forms of endometriosis are effective and may now be considered the "gold standard" of clinical care for women with endometriosis-related pain and infertility.

Women who desire pregnancy and whose disease is responsible for their symptoms of pain or infertility should have conservative operations.

Conservative operations attempt to remove all implants, resect adhesions, relieve pain, reduce the risk of recurrence and postoperative adhesions, and restore the involved organs to a normal anatomic and physiologic condition.

Radical ablative surgery is indicated mainly for pain that fail to respond to conservative treatment.

Procedures include oophorectomy, salpingo-oophorectomy, hysterectomy, appendicectomy, and excision of deeply infiltrating endometriosis possibly involving bowel resection.

Surgery must be carefully planned taking into consideration the patient's desire of fertility.

Polycystic Ovary Syndrome (PCOS)

PCOS is the most common manifestation of hormonal dysfunction in reproductive-age women today.

Treatment of polycystic ovaries should be targeted toward the patient's primary complaint, whether infertility, clinical signs of hyperandrogenism, or prolonged amenorrhea.

Treatment is focused on balancing the elevated circulating androgens and restoring the normal endocrine axis either via weight reduction or pharmacologic assistance.

Decreasing functional ovarian mass may diminish intra-ovarian androgen production and possibly encourage increased FSH levels.

This theory dates back to Stein and Leventhal's original work involving wedge resection of the ovary.

The technique, however, had been shown to be effective in as many as 90 % of reported cases.

Laparoscopic ovarian drilling also offers the benefit of altering the hormonal composite of PCOS patients after surgery.

There is often a reported decrease in serum LH, androgen concentration, and DHEA levels.

This reduction in the intra-ovarian androgen levels allows for the development of functional follicles.

Laparoscopic ovarian drilling is efficacious and carries with it the benefit of multiple ovulatory cycles, relatively short operative time, a decrease in spontaneous abortions, and a lowered risk of multiple gestations.

Selection of laparoscopic technique for management of PCOS should be carefully assessed as it has potential iatrogenic effects on the patient that may compromise the fertility, such as significant postoperative tubo-ovarian adhesions.

Ovarian Cystectomy

An ideal ovarian cystectomy consists of the removal of the intact cyst with limited trauma to the residual ovarian tissue.

Aspiration is recommended for functional cysts detected laparoscopically and confirmed by frozen section.

Cyst excision is preferred because thermal ablation does not destroy the entire cyst wall and the underlying ovarian cortex may be damaged by the heat.

The intact removal of a cyst 10 cm or larger is difficult laparoscopically.

Aspiration before removal of large cysts is practical.

The method that works best for endometriomas and mucinous cystadenomas involves the passage of a 5-mm trocar and sleeve into the cyst and then removed then the suction-irrigator is inserted into the cyst.

The aspirate is sent for cytologic examination, and the ovary is freed from adhesions to the lateral pelvic wall, uterus, or bowel.

The cyst and pelvis are irrigated continuously.

The most dependent portion of the cyst wall is opened, and the internal surface is inspected.

If excrescences or papillae are found, a biopsy specimen is sent for frozen section.

The capsule is stripped from the ovarian stroma using two grasping forceps and the suction-irrigator probe for traction and countertraction.

It is sent for histologic examination. Sealing blood vessels at the base of the capsule is done.

Tissue can be removed from the abdominal cavity by using one of the following techniques:

– Containment bags.

– Colpotomy.

– The cystic mass is brought to the surface of the abdominal incision, drained, and extracted similar to colpotomy.

The above method is not advisable for benign cystic teratomas that contain hair, as well as it may be time consuming and requires expert surgical technique.

For large teratomas (≥ 8 cm); the ovary is placed in the culde-sac next to a colpotomy.

Draining the cyst and removing its wall transvaginally lessen the risk of contamination and maintain a minimally invasive approach.

Compared with conventional laparoscopic cystectomy, there is less of a tendency to spill the contents and operative time is reduced.

Myomectomy

If the patient has a pedunculated fibroid, the stalk may be easily incised.

Excision of subserosal and intramural fibroids is more challenging.

The uterine incision is made with electrosurgery, and the myoma capsule is dissected.

A laparoscopic myoma screw may be helpful in providing traction during the dissection.

Electrosurgery, sharp dissection, and laser have been used successfully for myomectomy.

The irrigator-aspirator may be used for aquadissection and to maintain a clear surgical field.

Multiple myomata should be removed through a single uterine incision, if possible.

Venous bleeding can be managed with fulguration.

The myometrium should be closed with 0 or 2-0 absorbable suture; the serosa is closed with 4-0 suture.

Fibroid can be fragmented surgically or with an endoscopic morcellator and removed through large ports or through a colpotomy incision.

Indigo carmine dye can be injected into the endometrial cavity to evaluate its integrity after myomectomy.

Contraindications to laparoscopic myomectomy include diffuse disease, multiple myomata exceeding 5 cm, uterine size larger than 16 weeks, or a single myoma larger than 15 cm.

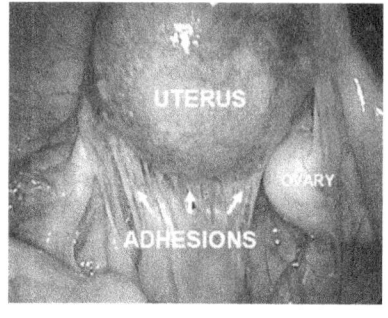

Pelvic Adhesions

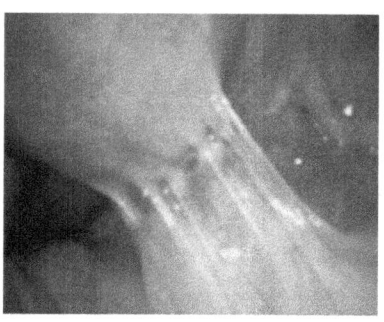

Lysis of Adhesions

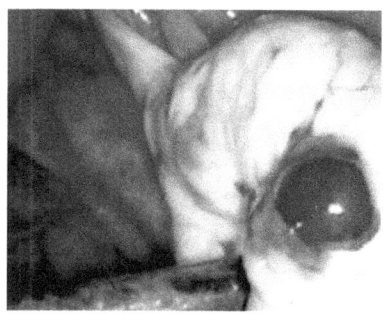

Ovarian Endometriosis

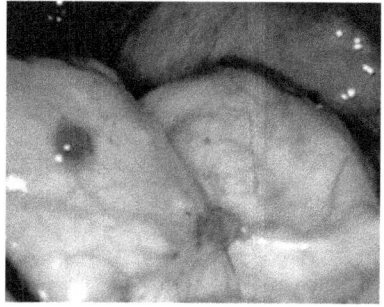

Rectosegmoid Endometriosis

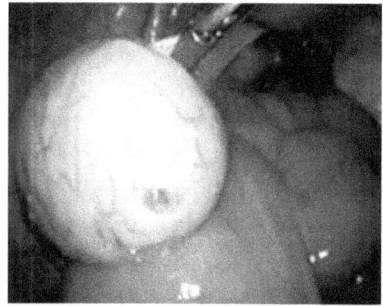

Polycystic Ovary

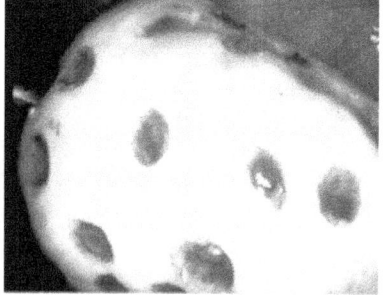

Ovarian Drilling

Laparoscopy: Indications

EQUIPMENT OF LAPAROSCOPY

Endoscopic surgery relies heavily not only on the skill of the surgeon but also on technology, much more than is the case with conventional surgery.

It is essential that the surgeon fully understands all aspects of the use of the equipment, from basic physical principles to how equipment is assembled and connected, from when and how to use a particular instrument, and what to do when it appears to be malfunctioning.

Insufflation Needles

Insufflation needle "Veress needle" is a hollow needle used to inflate the peritoneal cavity with CO_2 gas, before inserting the trocar and the laparoscope.

Traditionally, at the start of laparoscopy, gynecologists prefer to insufflate the abdomen with gas using Veress needle.

Disposable and reusable Veress needles consist of a blunt-tipped, spring-loaded inner stylet and a sharp outer needle.

A lateral hole on this stylet enables CO_2 gas to be delivered.

As the needle passes through the abdominal layers, the stylet retracts to allow penetration into the peritoneal cavity.

The absence of tissue resistance allows the blunt stylet to protrude intra-abdominally.

The disposable Veress needle has several added safety points, related mainly to the sharp tip of the outer needle and the smooth operation of the spring mechanism.

Laparoscopic Insufflator

To adequately observe the contents of the abdominal and pelvic cavity, the abdomen is distended with insufflated CO_2.

Laparoscopy requires delivering system capable of controlling intra-abdominal pressure rather than flow, and this should be set at 12-15 mmHg; to compensate for leakage when changing instrument and suction evacuation of smoke from electrodissection or laser.

A high pressure of up to 25 mmHg is acceptable during the set-up phase as this has the effect of increasing the distance between any trocar being inserted and bowel or large blood vessels, thereby in theory at least, reducing the risk of injury.

Some insufflators allow CO_2 to be warmed prior to insufflation and others have smoke traps, useful when doing CO_2 laser surgery.

This may help maintaining body temperature, decreasing risk of hypothermia, and reducing endoscope fogging.

Primary Trocars and Cannulas

Laparoscopic cannulas are hollow tubes with a valve or sealing mechanism at the proximal end.

Cannulas allow insertion of laparoscopic instruments into the peritoneal cavity while maintaining the pressure created by the distending gas.

The cannula may be fitted with a Luer-type port that allows attachment to tubing connected with the CO_2 insufflator.

Larger-diameter cannulas (8-12 mm) may be fitted with specialized valves that allow the insertion of smaller-diameter instruments without loss of intraperitoneal pressure.

The trocar is a longer instrument of slightly smaller diameter that is passed through the cannula, exposing its tip.

Most trocars have sharp tips, allowing penetration of the abdominal wall after a small skin incision.

Reusable and disposable trocars are constructed of a combination of metal and plastic.

All trocars have got a flapper or trumpet valve that is designed to prevent gas leakage as the laparoscope or other instruments are removed from the abdomen.

With reusable trocars, this mechanism creates friction on the laparoscope, making the trocar movable with the laparoscope, and thus leading to removal of the trocar from the abdominal cavity and a loss of pneumoperitoneum.

When the spring is removed from the valve, there is less friction and that problem can be avoided.

Another approach to improving the safety of primary trocar insertion is the observing or optical trocar.

The trocar-cannula assembly is passed through tissue layers to enter the operative space under direct vision from a 10 mm or a 5 mm $0°$ laparoscope placed into the trocar.

A fiberglass optic-equipped safety needle has been developed for visually controlled access in laparoscopic procedures.

This device can allow immediate diagnosis of small bowel perforation by endoscopy.

Various disposable trocar tips are available.

Spring-loaded safety shields retract into the cannula as the trocar is inserted into the abdomen.

This exposes the sharp trocar for entry and automatically releases the plastic shield inside the peritoneal cavity to cover the sharp tip and protect intra-abdominal organs.

Another trocar uses the same principle as the Veress needle.

Secondary Trocars and Cannulas

Secondary cannulas are necessary to perform most diagnostic and operative laparoscopic procedures.

Most currently available disposable ancillary cannulas are identical to those designed for insertion of the primary cannula, however, simple cannulas without safety sheaths and insufflations ports are sufficient.

Reusable and disposable accessory trocars and sleeves come in a variety of lengths and range in diameter from 2 to 30 mm; the most common size is 5 mm.

Some are threaded and are screwed into the abdominal wall, making them relatively immobile during manipulation.

The use of "fascial screws" is associated with an increased incidence of omental and bowel herniation after laparoscopy.

The Laparoscope

The laparoscope allows one to view the abdominal and pelvic cavities and is the most important piece of equipment.

It comes in a variety of diameters (2-12 mm) and angles of view (0°-90°); with direct 10 mm, 0° diagnostic laparoscope and 11 mm, 0° operative laparoscopes preferable.

The most commonly used laparoscopes are straight diagnostic and angled operative laparoscopes.

Operating laparoscopes have an additional operating channel for instruments or lasers but are less popular.

Most gynecologists prefer to use a multipuncture approach with instruments inserted through ancillary ports.

Endoscopes are either rigid or flexible.

Flexible scopes rely on many fiberoptic bundles.

As the image is magnified, so are the bundles, making the ends of the bundles visible along with the image.

LAPAROSCOPY: Equipment

The scopes are relatively fragile, and small cracks allow water to seep through the lens and distort the image.

With a Hopkins rod lens system, the shaft of the laparoscope contains quartz rods with concave ends that provide excellent clarity.

This type of lens is rarely dislodged during handling.

With a videoscope (camera and scope together), either there will be a focus control on the scope or the focus will occur automatically inside the camera.

The image is magnified and appears larger on the monitor.

Light Sources and Light Cord

Illumination is primarily a function of power of the light and the light transmission properties of the light lead, but is also influenced by the size and tissue properties of what is being illuminated.

For instance, laparoscopy requires a brighter light to sufficiently illuminate a larger cavity at a greater distance, and the same is true in the presence of bleeding as blood absorbs light.

Older tungsten and metal halide light sources have been replaced by more powerful xenon generators.

Light leads are of two types: fiber optic or liquid.

The fiber optic leads are more common because they are cheaper, but the fibers are prone to breaking with gradual deterioration in light transmission.

Rough handling (e.g. kinking, knotting, or tight rolling) should be avoided as this will tend to damage the delicate light fibers.

The state of the fibers is easily checked by aiming at one end at a light and looking at the other end for dark areas.

Liquid light cables transmit more light and are more durable than fiber optic cables, but they are more expensive, produce more heat, and can be irreversibly damaged if the outer casing is punctured.

Suction-Irrigator Probe and Hydrodissection Pump

Suction-irrigation system is an absolute requirement for operative procedures.

Not only it can be used to aspirate blood and clean the pelvis, but ovarian cysts can be deflated, ectopic pregnancies sucked out and hydrodissection used in difficult cases.

Forceps

Atraumatic stabilization of structures is important in many procedures, and several types of forceps are available for this purpose.

Atraumatic and grasping forceps with jaws are available in sizes from 3 to 10 mm.

The preferred type is medium sized, with a rounded tip and serrated jaws.

Scissors

Scissors are curved, straight, or hooked.

Some have electrical adaptor so that they can be combined with unipolar or bipolar electrocoagulation.

Scissors are inserted into the secondary trocar under direct observation to avoid injury to pelvic structures.

Biopsy Forceps

Biopsy forceps can sample suspected endometrial implants, ovarian lesions, and peritoneum.

The forceps jaws should be sharp and overlap when closed to avoid tearing tissue and causing unnecessary bleeding.

Electrosurgical Generator and Bipolar Forceps

The primary instrument used for hemostasis during operative laparoscopy is the bipolar electrocoagulator.

The modern generator safely and reliably delivers a high-frequency current at low voltage.

It can be used in one of three modalities:

– Bipolar,

– Monopolar cutting (including pure cut and blended cut), and

– Monopolar coagulation (including desiccation, fulguration and spray).

Bipolar coagulation is often used in laparoscopy; the bipolar circuit has the lowest voltage, hence, it is the safest when working in the pelvis.

Several types of bipolar forceps are available.

Fine tips are used for coagulating small blood vessels during delicate operations involving the tubes, bowel, or ureter.

Flatter jaws are appropriate for use on large blood vessels or pedicles, including the uterine artery and the infundibulopelvic ligaments.

The main advantage of bipolar energy to monopolar energy is more controlled spread of energy because energy travels only in the small space between the two jaws.

Vessel-Sealing Systems

The ever present need to facilitate advanced laparoscopic procedures has brought about the invention of new modalities for achieving hemostasis.

Beside titanium clips and laparoscopic stapling devices, there are two other modalities: bipolar vessel-sealing devices and ultrasonic energy.

Laser and Laser Equipment

Unlike electrosurgery, lasers are by no means essential for effective endoscopic surgery as there is no evidence that they produce a better end result.

However, under certain conditions, as dissecting near vital structures, lasers may represent a safer surgical modality because thermal spread tends to be less.

Lasers tend to be less efficient at hemostasis than diathermy.

Several different lasers are available for endoscopy, but of these CO_2, Nd: YAG (neodymium: yttrium-aluminum-garnet), argon and KTP (potassium titanyl phosphate) lasers tend to be used for laparoscopy and Nd: YAG for hysteroscopy.

Uterine Manipulators

Safe, effective endoscopy requires adequate mobilization and stabilization of the uterus and associated organs.

Various combinations of uterine sounds, cannulas, and dilators are available.

The Camera

The camera includes camera head with its cable and camera controller.

The cable is plugged into the camera controller.

The lens on the medical camera is called a coupler.

The coupler screws onto the camera head and is available in several sizes that magnify the image.

A 24-mm coupler will produce a larger image on the monitor than will a 20-mm coupler

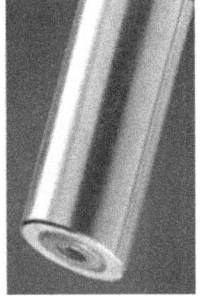 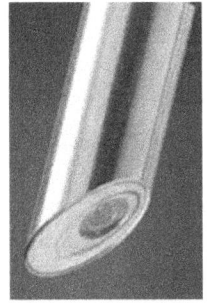 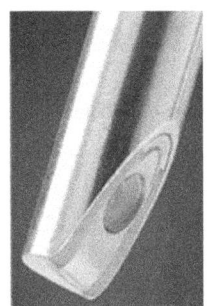

Straight and Angled Laparoscopes

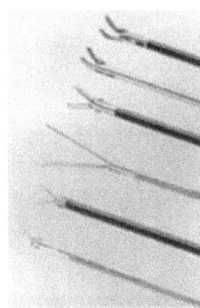 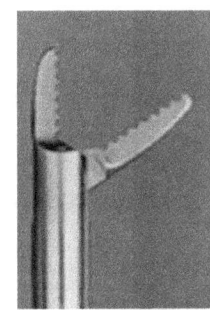 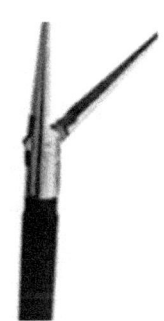

Laparoscopic Grasping Forceps

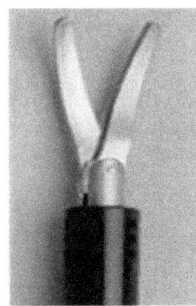 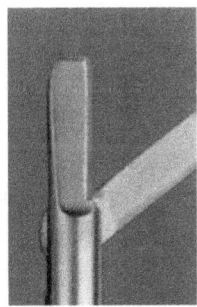 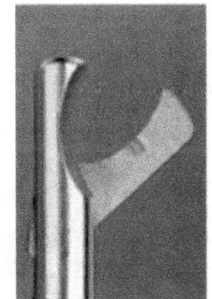

Laparoscopic Scissors

Laparoscopy: Equipment

RELEVANT ANATOMY

Anterior abdominal wall anatomy should receive special attention prior to laparoscopy because many laparoscopic complications result from trocar placement.

Abdominal Scars

Previous surgery is associated with a greater than 20% risk of adhesions of bowel or omentum to the anterior abdominal wall.

For this reason, many laparoscopists adjust their techniques in these patients to minimize the risk of bowel injury.

Of special concern are incisional scars immediately adjacent to the umbilicus because bowel adherent underneath the umbilicus may be at risk for injury.

Although Pfannenstiel and abdominal incisions distant to the umbilicus may also be associated with adhesions, in many laparoscopists' experiences, these incisions appear to represent less of a risk than incisions near the umbilicus.

In addition to location, the width and depth of the scar should be evaluated because a wide or retracted scar may suggest that a postoperative wound infection had occurred.

Common wisdom dictates that postoperative infections may be associated with an increased risk of intra-abdominal adhesion formation, although no data are available to support this observation.

If the dome of the bladder is involved in the infectious process, it may cause progression of the bladder dome higher behind the anterior abdominal wall, thus increasing the risk of bladder injury at the time of suprapubic trocar placement.

Abdominal Wall Thickness

Although abdominal thickness correlates with patient weight, short stature or truncal obesity may increase abdominal wall thickness out of proportion to patient weight.

Routine evaluation of the abdominal wall prior to laparoscopy is important because the success of trocar insertion may depend on altering the technique based on abdominal wall thickness.

Umbilicus

The umbilicus should be examined for signs of umbilical hernia.

Techniques for trocar insertion should be adjusted, and closure of the defect should be considered.

In the absence of incarcerated bowel, the skin over the hernia can be carefully incised and the peritoneal cavity entered using an open technique.

Closure of a small defect can be performed with interrupted sutures at the completion of the laparoscopic procedure.

Abdominal Wall Vessels

The anterior abdominal wall contains 2 sets of bilateral vessels: the superficial and the inferior (deep) epigastric vessels.

These arteries originate from the femoral and external iliac arteries, respectively, and are accompanied by a large vein in most cases.

Immediately above the symphysis pubis, they are both located an average of 5.5 cm from the midline and course slightly more laterally at points more cephalad.

In order to avoid injuring these vessels during lateral trocar placement, the superficial vessels should be visualized by transillumination and the inferior vessels should be laparoscopically visualized whenever possible.

The use of conical trocars can also decrease the risk of injury to these vessels.

TECHNIQUE OF LAPAROSCOPY

Preoperative Preparation

Careful preoperative evaluation and preparation of the patient optimizes the operative outcome and decreases the incidence of complications and injuries.

Complete patient's medical history, taking into account prior surgical history, should be taken and understood, as well as performing thorough physical examination.

Laboratory and radiologic studies may be indicated in patients with known health problems.

The preoperative discussion should include a description of the planned operation, possible outcome and results, possible complications, and the surgeon's experience in doing that particular procedure.

It may be helpful to compare risks and recovery with the same procedure performed via.

The patient needs to be aware that any endoscopic operation may have to be converted to laparotomy; that bowel, bladder and ureteric injury are accepted risks with laparoscopy, and uterine perforation and fluid overload with hysteroscopy.

Then a signed informed consent for endoscopy must be obtained.

Laparoscopic Procedure

The anaesthesiology team and circulating nurses coordinate the patient's transfer onto the operating table.

The operative site is cleansed and shaved preoperatively by an operating room nurse.

Proper positioning of the patient is essential for patient safety, comfort of the operator and optimal visualization of the pelvic organs.

LAPAROSCOPY: Technique

The patient is placed in lithotomy position after induction of endotracheal anaesthesia (to minimize risk of aspiration).

Once the patient is positioned, her abdomen, perineum and vagina are prepared with a suitable bactericidal solution and a Foley catheter is inserted.

The patient is draped to expose the abdomen and the perineum.

Bimanual examination is done to confirm the size, position and mobility of the uterus as well as any adnexal pathology.

Both the hysteroscope and the laparoscope are connected to the light sources and cameras.

Diagnostic hysteroscopy, if needed, is done at this step.

Sometimes it is indicated for patients undergoing diagnostic or operative laparoscopy.

The first Mayo stand is moved out of the way and all the setup tables are brought close to the operating table.

The uterus is sounded and a uterine manipulator is inserted into the cervical os to manipulate the uterus and for chromopertubation.

Peritoneal access can be established by placing a cannula or port in the abdominal wall before inserting the trocar and the laparoscope.

Veress Needle and Primary Trocar Insertion

The optimal location for the Veress needle and primary trocar is the umbilicus because the skin is attached to the fascial layer and anterior parietal peritoneum with no intervening subcutaneous fat or muscle.

This site is the shortest distance between the skin and the peritoneal cavity even in obese patients.

Modification of the site sometimes is done in patients who have an enlarged uterus caused by a uterine leiomyoma, pregnancy or for para-aortic lymph node dissection, the primary trocar is inserted approximately 4 to 6 cm above the umbilicus.

Before the needle is inserted, the base of the umbilicus is elevated by a skin hook or Allis clamp and a vertical cutaneous incision (better cosmetically) is made large enough to accommodate the primary trocar.

The surgeon and assistants apply countertraction by grasping the skin and fat on each side of the umbilicus with a towel clip.

The Veress needle, held at the shaft, is directed toward the sacral promontory.

Traditionally, the angle of insertion of the insufflation needle, the primary trocar, and the cannula, is approximately 45°, accomplished best while the patient is completely horizontal, and the operating table is all the way down to maximize the surgeon's upper body control during insertion.

Insertion of the needle and cannula is aided by an understanding of the normal underlying anatomy, especially the location of the larger retroperitoneal vessels.

A safety zone exists inferior to the sacral promontory in the area bounded cephalad by the bifurcation of the aorta, posteriorly by the sacrum, and laterally by the iliac vessels.

In women placed in the Trendelenburg position, the great vessels are situated more cephalad and anterior, making them more vulnerable to injury unless appropriate adjustments are made in the angle of insertion.

Gynecologists have generally favored a closed technique; preinflating the peritoneal cavity with CO_2 through a hollow insufflation needle.

Verification of Intraperitoneal Location

First, the patency of the needle should be checked before it is inserted.

LAPAROSCOPY: Technique

Failure to achieve and maintain a suitable pneumoperitoneum predisposes the patient to complications.

Correct needle placement is verified by the "hanging drop" technique or the syringe test.

In "hanging drop" method, a drop of saline is placed on the hub of the Veress needle after insertion through the abdominal wall; and the abdominal wall is lifted to create negative pressure within the abdomen, drawing the drop of fluid into the needle.

Alternatively, a 10-ml syringe with normal saline is attached to the Veress needle and aspiration verifies the absence of bowel contents or blood.

The saline is injected into the peritoneal cavity, and if the needle placement is correct, the fluid cannot be withdrawn because it is dispersed intraperitoneally.

Pneumoperitoneum

A pneumoperitoneum is a prerequisite for laparoscopic observation, exposure and intraperitoneal manipulations.

The pressure recorded within the abdomen initially should be no greater than 9 or 10 mmHg.

If higher pressures are recorded, the needle has been placed improperly.

The surgeon should use palpable abdominal distension and the pressure reading rather than the volume of gas insufflated because they more accurately reflect the adequacy of the pneumoperitoneum.

After insertion of the trocars, the intra-abdominal pressure should be preset between 12 and 16 mmHg during the operative procedure.

Higher pressures for long periods may cause subcutaneous emphysema.

Pneumoperitoneum reduces the proximity of the abdominal wall to the spine and the potential for damage to bowel and vessels.

Placement of Accessory Trocars

Accessory trocars are used for most gynecologic laparoscopy procedures.

After identifying the epigastric vessels by transillumination and intraperitoneal observation, 1-3 secondary trocars are placed, depending on the procedure and the number of trocars required for the operation.

The trocars are placed either in the midline, 3 cm above the symphysis pubis, or laterally, approximately 8 cm from the midline and 8 cm above the symphysis pubis to avoid the inferior epigastric vessels, which is located approximately 5.5 cm from the midline.

Insertion of the trocar and removal of the sleeves are performed under direct laparoscopic visualization while observing for signs of hemorrhage.

If the trocar is larger than 8 mm, the fascia is closed with suture after removal of the sleeve to reduce risk of hernia.

Pelvic Exploration

The initial phase of laparoscopy is to identify anatomic landmarks and approach the female pelvis systematically and anatomically.

The examination should begin with a survey of the midline structures and progress to the right and left adnexa.

This helps to assessand document the extent of the disease.

In the beginning, the upper abdomen, including the abdominal wall, liver, gallbladder, and diaphragm, is examined for any abnormality that could contribute to the patient's symptoms.

The intestine and omentum are examined for any injury that could have happened during insertion of laparoscopic instruments.

Then the laparoscope is returned to view the pelvic cavity.

LAPAROSCOPY: Technique

The characteristics of the bladder, ureters, colon, rectum, uterosacral ligaments, and major blood vessels are noted.

The appendix is inspected for endometriosis.

Then, the right adnexa are assessed after the posterior cul-de-sac is filled with irrigation fluid.

The fimbriae are lifted, and the posterior aspect of the ovary and the ovarian fossa are evaluated.

The ureter is seen, and its direction is traced from the pelvic brim to the bladder.

The uterus is anteverted, and the uterosacral ligaments, posterior cul-de-sac, and rectum are examined.

The patient is placed in a 30° Trendelenburg position to allow the surgeon to push the small bowel into the upper abdomen to aid in viewing the posterior cul-de-sac.

The rectosigmoid colon and its folds are evaluated, and after the rectosigmoid is pushed laterally, the left and right pararectal areas are examined.

Then the left ovary and tube are evaluated in the same manner.

In the presence of extensive adhesions, this technique is modified.

The gynecologist ascertains the approximate location of the normal structures, assesses the type of adhesions, plans the procedure, and decides whether the procedure is to be done by laparoscopy or laparotomy.

This decision depends on the abnormalities, the time needed to correct them, and the surgeon's experience.

Ending the Operation

At the end of the operation, chromopertubation is done in all infertility patients intraoperatively.

The patient's position is changed from Trendelenburg to horizontal to allow fluid from the upper abdomen to collect in the pelvic cavity.

The entire peritoneal cavity is irrigated copiously with isotonic fluid, usually lactated Ringer's solution, and inspected for blood clots, pieces of adhesions, cyst wall, endometriosis implants, and bleeding.

Bleeding points are identified and coagulated with bipolar forceps.

Because the intra-abdominal pressure created by the pneumoperitoneum can tamponade bleeding from small vessels, the gas is evacuated temporarily and the operative sites are inspected for bleeding before the abdominal cavity is reinsufflated.

The presence of clear irrigating fluid confirms adequate hemostasis.

The ancillary ports should be removed under direct vision followed by deflation of the abdomen via the port used for the optic.

By keeping the laparoscope inside the cannula as it is being withdrawn, it is possible to check that this port site is not bleeding and has not caught a loop of bowel or omentum.

The procedure is concluded by evacuating the CO_2 from the abdomen.

Release of Pneumoperitoneum

The CO_2 used to distend the abdomen is evacuated to reduce postoperative shoulder pain caused by gas trapped under the diaphragm.

The patient is put in a straight, supine position as the gas escapes from the umbilical and suprapubic trocars.

Suprapubic trocars are removed under low pneumoperitoneal pressure to search for possible inferior epigastric vessel injury.

The umbilical trocar is removed, and the skin incisions are inspected for bleeding.

Except for patients in whom Interceed is applied, 300 to 400 ml of lactated Ringer's solution is left in the abdominal cavity to aid in displacing the gas and possibly to decrease postoperative adhesions.

Since this procedure was used, the prevalence of postoperative shoulder pain has decreased.

Closure of Incisions

A laparoscopic procedure is not complete until all port incisions have been closed.

The trocar incisions are closed using Steri-Strips or inverted subcutaneous 4-0 polyglactin sutures.

Incisions made for trocars larger than 5mm are closed in layers, especially in older or thin women, because failure to close the fascia has been associated with small bowel strangulation and hernia.

Several instruments, including the J-needle and the Carter-Thomason needle, have been developed to allow for fascial and peritoneal closure of the trocar site incisions under direct observation.

When the procedure is completed, instruments are handled carefully so that laparoscopes and other delicate equipment are not damaged.

The disposable equipment is discarded, and the reusable instruments are given to the circulating nurses for cleaning.

The patient's legs are lowered and her abdomen is washed thoroughly.

Postoperative Care

Before the operation, the patient is provided with postoperative instructions to prepare for the postoperative experience.

After the operation, the gynecologist sees the patient in the extended recovery room to explain the operative findings and the expected postoperative course.

LAPAROSCOPY: Technique

For any procedure, pain may be perceived as slightly worse on the day following the procedure but should improve after this point.

Likewise, the incision should appear healthy and become almost painless within the first week.

Progressive resolution of symptoms is expected 3-7 days after any gynecologic laparoscopic procedure.

The most common complaint after laparoscopic procedures is shoulder pain referred from the collection of CO_2 under the diaphragm.

Generally, it resolves within 48 hours post operatively.

Resting on the abdomen with pillows under it may be helpful.

Elevating the lower pelvis also alleviates this pain.

Nausea and vomiting most likely are related to intra-abdominal CO_2 and the narcotics frequently used perioperatively.

Usually these symptoms respond to parenteral antiemetic medication.

Occasionally, a patient develops hypotension unrelated to blood loss.

These patients are cured promptly after a bolus of intravenous fluid is given.

Postoperative incisional pain is usually mild and is managed by using a heating pad and analgesics.

Patients who undergo extensive intra-abdominal procedures may have severe visceral pain.

Narcotic or non-steroidal anti-inflammatory agents are needed in addition to a heating pad.

Persistent pain for more than a few hours after release from the hospital requires that the patient be examined.

When large amounts of isotonic fluid are left in the abdomen, the patient tends to drain pinkish fluid through the abdominal puncture wounds.

This ceases within 24 to 48 hours; reassurance of the patient only is needed.

Probably the most concerning postoperative symptom is worsening abdominal pain, especially in the presence of distension.

Unfortunately, signs of an occult injury of bowel or bladder may take hours or days to develop.

Herniation manifests as severe abdominal pain accompanied by signs of bowel obstruction.

An unusual cause of abdominal pain after laparoscopy can be an entrapped incisional hernia.

It is not related to herniation through a fascial defect; it can be herniated bowel through the peritoneum into the preperitoneal space and got entrapped.

Before discharge, patients are given prescriptions for pain medications as needed, routine postoperative instructions and should be instructed to contact their physician if any deviation from the normal expected postoperative course occurred.

Follow-up

In the absence of complications, the patient should be able to return to full activity within 72 hours after most gynecologic laparoscopic procedures other than hysterectomy (takes 2-3 weeks).

Because complete healing of fascial defects takes several weeks, the patient should avoid lifting anything heavier than 15 pounds for the first month.

Follow-up office visits in patients without complications are usually scheduled 2-4 weeks after surgery.

LAPAROSCOPY: Technique

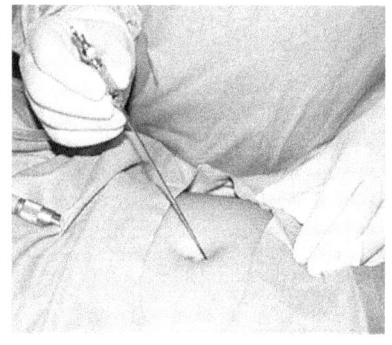

Veress Needle Insertion   Primary Trocar Insertion

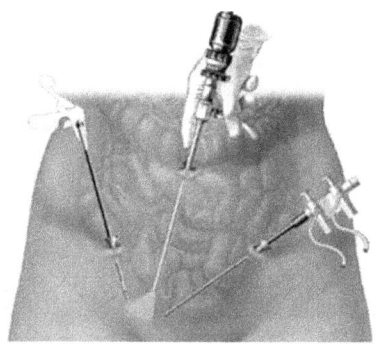
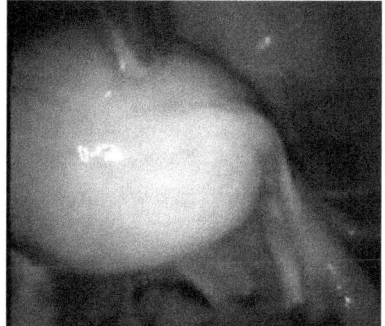

Accessory Trocars Insertion   Pelvic Exploration

Laparoscopy: Technique

COMPLICATIONS OF LAPAROSCOPY

Laparoscopic procedures can be complicated by infections, trauma, or hemorrhage, as well as by problems associated with anesthetic use.

The incidence of infection is lower than with procedures performed by laparotomy.

Conversely, problems associated with visualization in conjunction with the change in anatomic perspective may increase the risk of damage to blood vessels or vital structures such as the bowel, ureter, or bladder.

Intraoperative Complications

Complications of Anesthesia

Increased intra-abdominal pressure caused by pneumoperitoneum, absorption of CO_2 gas or fluid, and the Trendelenburg position concern anesthesiologists.

The potential risks of general anesthesia include hypoventilation, esophageal intubation, gastroesophageal reflux, bronchospasm, hypotension, narcotic overdose, cardiac arrhythmias, and cardiac arrest.

A vasovagal reaction and cardiac arrhythmias developing from CO_2 absorption are avoided by administering atropine preoperatively.

The Trendelenburg position, in combination with the increased intraperitoneal pressure provided by pneumoperitoneum, places greater pressure on the diaphragm; increasing the risk of hypoventilation, hypercarbia, and metabolic acidosis.

Trendelenburg position, combined with anesthetic agents that relax the esophageal sphincter, promotes regurgitation of gastric content, which in turn can lead to aspiration, bronchospasm, pneumonitis, and pneumonia.

Fluid overload and high molecular weight dextran used as a distension medium for hysteroscopy are circumvented by accurately measuring input and output.

Pulmonary edema is a rare complication of absorbing crystalloid irrigating fluid during laparoscopy.

Lavage with large volumes of room temperature irrigation fluid can be associated with hypothermia, so the fluid should be warmed or a heating blanket should be used.

The use of warmed irrigation fluid decreased the drop in core temperature associated with laparoscopy.

Reconditioning laparoscopic gas by filtering, heating, and hydrating the gas may reduce or eliminate laparoscopically induced hypothermia, shortening recovery room stay and reducing postoperative pain.

Gas Embolism

Because CO_2 is used to create the pneumoperitoneum in laparoscopic procedures, gas embolization is an uncommon but very serious complication.

Embolization is usually caused by inadvertent placement of the Veress needle into a major vessel (of the venous system) during attempts to insufflate the abdominal cavity with CO_2.

To avoid this complication, the operator must verify intraperitoneal placement of Veress needle prior to insufflation.

Clinical signs include decreased end-tidal CO_2, decreased oxygen saturation, a loud mill-wheel murmur, severe hypotension, and possible cardiac arrest.

Treatment includes immediately stopping insufflation, removing the needle, placing the patient in the left lateral decubitus position, administering 100% oxygen, and giving cardiac support.

The gas embolism may be broken up with external cardiac massage, but definitive treatment is placement of a central line for aspiration of the gas from the right side of the heart and from the pulmonary vasculature.

Procedural Failures

It is better to complete a procedure by laparotomy than to risk injury to the patient or be forced to proceed with an emergency laparotomy because of a complication.

The possibility of complications is increased during the insertion of the Veress needle and primary and secondary trocars in patients with multiple previous laparotomies, those with a body mass index >30, and very thin patients.

Bowel preparation is recommended if there is a risk of bowel injury.

Veress needle and trocar insertion is modified in the presence of a large pelvic mass.

Electrosurgical Injuries

Complications of electrosurgery occur secondary to thermal injury from unintended or inappropriate use of the active electrode, current diversion to an undesirable path, and injury at the site of the dispersive electrode.

The first response to electrosurgical equipment failure should never be to increase the current.

Even properly functioning equipment can result in injury.

If the foot pedal is accidentally depressed, tissue adjacent to the electrode will be traumatized.

Potential sites of injury include the bowel, ureter, or, if the electrode lies on the abdomen, the skin.

Injury from direct extension of thermal effect can occur when the zone of vaporization or coagulation extends to large blood vessels or vital structures such as the bladder, ureter, or bowel.

The diagnosis of direct thermal visceral injury may be difficult.

If unintended activation of the electrode occurs, nearby intraperitoneal structures should be evaluated carefully.

Thermal injury that is recognized at the time of laparoscopy should be managed immediately, taking into consideration the potential extent of the zone of coagulative necrosis.

The diagnosis of visceral thermal injury is often delayed until signs and symptoms of fistula or peritonitis appear.

Because these complications may not manifest until 2 to 10 days after surgery, patients should be advised to report any postoperative fever or increasing abdominal pain.

Bleeding

Uncontrolled bleeding and hemorrhage are the cause of most emergency laparotomies.

Bleeding occurs during sharp dissection of adhesions, transaction of vessels during laser excision or dissection, and rough handling of tissues.

Lacerations of the oviduct, mesosalpinx, and infundibulopelvic ligament can bleed profusely.

Distorted anatomy is an important compounding factor in many cases of major retroperitoneal vascular injury.

When pressure gradients return to normal, bleeding into the retroperitoneal space may begin, eventually leading to hematoma and hypovolemic shock.

All exposed vessels should be evaluated at the end of the procedure with the patient supine and intra-abdominal pressure reduced.

Blood clots in the pelvic side wall should be evacuated before complete hemostasis is confirmed.

Small Bowel Injuries

Small bowel injuries occur if the bowel is immobilized by adhesions.

The bowel can be injured during insertion of the Veress needle or trocar, bowel manipulation, or enterolysis.

Electrosurgery and stray laser beams can result in unrecognized thermal injuries to the bowel. Injury to the gastrointestinal tract is a serious complication.

Whether discovered intraoperatively or postoperatively, small bowel injuries may necessitate a laparotomy to avoid serious morbidity and even mortality.

Large Bowel Injuries

Colon entry is a major complication, particularly if the bowel is unprepared or the injury is not recognized.

Even small perforations, such as those from the Veress needle, require attention because the high bacterial concentration of minor leaks can cause infection and abscess formation.

Factors that contribute to an increased risk of large bowel injuries include:

– Failure to establish an adequate pneumoperitoneum;

– The use of dull trocars that require excessive force;

– Uncontrolled, sudden entry of sharp instruments; and

– Gastric distension.

Uterine Injuries

Complications involving the uterus may include cervical lacerations or uterine perforation from sounding the uterus, and the use of a uterine dilator or uterine manipulator.

Bladder Injuries

Vesical injury is rare and occurs in patients who have had laparotomies or whose bladders are not empty.

Under these conditions, trocars, uterine anteverters, and blunt instruments can perforate or lacerate the bladder and electrosurgery and lasers can cause thermal injury.

Ureteral Injuries

Knowledge of the ureter's path through the pelvis and the vulnerable points is the key to preventing injuries.

The intrapelvic segment of the ureter is near the broad ligament, ovaries, and uterosacral ligaments and injuries occur in those areas.

The ureter is at risk during laparoscopic surgery when the cardinal ligament is dissected and divided below the uterine vessels.

Endometriosis and severe pelvic adhesions can thicken the peritoneum, obscuring the location of the ureter, especially near the uterosacral ligaments.

Ureteral injury can occur in the course of sharp dissection of an ovary adherent to the pelvic side wall; uterosacral transaction; ligation, transaction, and coagulation of the uterine arteries; removal of endometriotic implants or fibrosis from the ureter; and attempts to control bleeding vessels.

Postoperative Complications

Bleeding

Hemostasis that appears adequate before closure because of the Trendelenburg position, high intra-abdominal pressures, and relative hypotension may change once the patient resumes an upright position.

If the patient does not respond to intravenous hydration, a repeat hematocrit may suggest hemorrhage and a physical exam may reveal abdominal distension.

Nerve Injuries

Peripheral nerve injury is usually related either to poor positioning of the patient or to excessive pressure exerted by the surgeons.

Nerve injury may also occur as a result of the surgical dissection.

Common postoperative neurologic syndromes include sciatic nerve injury, brachial palsy (shoulder-hand syndrome), and perineal nerve palsy.

Allowing the buttocks to protrude too far off the end of the operating table may cause back injury.

In the extremities, the trauma may be direct, such as when the common peroneal nerve is compressed against the stirrups.

The femoral nerve or the sciatic nerve or its branches may be overstretched and damaged by excessive flexion or external rotation of the hips.

Most injuries to peripheral nerves resolve spontaneously.

Pain

Many patients still complain of moderate abdominal and shoulder pain during the first 48 to 72 hours postoperatively.

The CO_2 commonly used for insufflation is a peritoneal irritant.

Intraoperatively, this irritation can manifest as a vasovagal reaction.

Postoperatively, residual gas accumulates under the diaphragm, thus irritating it, and the pain is referred to the shoulder.

Warming the insufflation CO_2 gas reduces postoperative pain.

Infection

Postoperative infection is unusual after laparoscopic procedures, although the risk appears to be higher after prolonged, intricate procedures.

Most infections are limited to skin or stitch abscesses and require incision and drainage.

Urinary tract infections can be caused by instrumentation or asymptomatic bacteria.

Incisional Hernia

Herniation of the omentum or small bowel at the umbilical incision site has been reported with 5-mm or larger trocars.

Patients at increased risk are those who are very thin (especially the elderly), those with chronic coughs, and those with a history of hernias.

Incisional hernias, although infrequent, mostly occur in sites where trocars 10 mm in diameter or larger were used.

Vaginal Cuff Dehiscence

Vaginal vault rupture with intestinal herniation is a postoperative complication of total hysterectomy.

Mortality

Death, although extremely rare following minimally invasive surgical procedures, has been reported.

It is more commonly associated with unrecognized trauma to the intestinal tract with ensuing sequelae. It also has been reported in association with major vascular trauma.

CONTRAINDICATIONS OF LAPAROSCOPY

While having great advantages over traditional surgeries, laparoscopy may not be appropriate in some patients.

However, improvement in laparoscopic skills and experience, combined with the availability of the proper instruments, has reduced the number of conditions that were previously considered absolute contraindications for laparoscopy to relative contraindications.

Obesity

In obese women, every aspect of laparoscopy becomes more difficult and potentially more risky.

Placement of laparoscopic instruments and many intra-abdominal procedures become more difficult probably due to:

- Restricted operative field secondary to retroperitoneal fat deposits in the pelvic sidewalls,

- Increased volume of bowel, and decreased elevation of a heavier anterior abdominal wall by the pneumoperitoneum, and

- The inability to place many patients who are obese in steep Trendelenburg position because of ventilation considerations.

Multiple Abdominal Operations

The risk of adhesions of omentum and/or bowel to the anterior abdominal wall after previous abdominal surgery is great.

As laparoscopy requires the insertion of sharp instruments into the abdominal cavity, a reasonable assumption is that previous surgery would increase risk of bowel injury; thus, strategies have been developed to decrease bowel injury.

The most common of these strategies is the use of an open technique for laparoscopic trocar placement.

Age

Older patients are at increased risk of having concomitant diseases that affect their perioperative morbidity and mortality.

Probably the most important consideration is age-associated increase in cardiovascular disease.

Intraoperative cardiac stress related to anesthesia and the surgery itself may result in sudden cardiac decompensation based on arrhythmia, ischemia, or infarct.

Patients with class IV cardiac disease suffer adverse effects from pneumoperitoneum and Trendelenburg position, even for relatively short procedures.

Patients with class III cardiac disease can safely undergo procedures lasting <30 minutes.

Of special importance is that the vast majority of patients experience some degree of hypothermia during laparoscopy.

In older patients, even mild degrees of hypothermia may increase the risk of cardiac arrhythmia and prolong recovery time.

Bowel Perforation with Generalized Peritonitis

In patients with generalized peritonitis, the bowel is frequently matted and adherent to the abdominal wall.

However, laparoscopy was found to be safe and effective in the diagnosis and treatment of patients with peritonitis.

Laparoscopic treatment was practical in a patient who had an appendicular and gastroduodenal perforation.

Hypovoleminc Shock

Hemoperitoneum in an unstable patient has been considered a contraindication because the bleeding source may be difficult to find and treat laparoscopically.

However, laparoscopy offers many theoretical advantages for the immediate diagnosis and management of a patient presenting with hemodynamic instability and suspected active intra-abdominal bleeding caused by an ectopic pregnancy or a bleeding hemorrhagic corpus luteum.

These features include superior observation of the entire abdominal cavity, decreased intra-abdominal bleeding because of compression by the creation of a pneumoperitoneum, and ability to control the source of bleeding effectively with minimal tissue damage.

Intestinal Obstruction

Intestinal obstruction and bowel distension are associated with an increased risk of perforation.

Although laparoscopy is less invasive than laparotomy, bowel obstruction not relieved by conservative decompression techniques may require laparotomy.

Pregnancy

Intrauterine pregnancy >16 weeks and large intra-abdominal mass (higher than the equivalent of a 16 weeks pregnancy) have the risk of trauma during the insertion of trocars and cannulae.

Cancer

Laparoscopic surgery is contraindicated in advanced malignancies.

EFFICACY OF LAPAROSCOPY

Advantages

– Small abdominal incisions are better cosmetically, in addition to rapid postoperative recovery and early mobilization, thus minimizing the risk of DVT and pulmonary embolism and decreased incidence of other prolonged recumbency complications as constipation, urinary tract infections and depression.

– Early return of gastrointestinal activity due to less manipulation of the bowel during surgery, which results in fewer postoperative adhesions and intestinal obstruction.

– Shorter hospitalization time and prompt return to regular life.

– Fewer incidence of incisional hernia because of markedly smaller port of entry.

– Future fertility is not compromised and in some cases may be improved with laparoscopic treatment.

Disadvantages

– Exposure of the operative field can be reduced.

– Small instruments are required and can be used only through fixed ports.

– The ability to manipulate the pelvic viscera is limited.

– The caliber of the suture required may be larger than otherwise desired.

– In many cases, the cost of hospitalization increases, despite a shortened stay, because of prolonged operating room time and the use of more expensive surgical equipment and supplies.

– In some patients, there is an increased risk of complications, which can be attributed to the innate limitations of laparoscopy, the level of surgical expertise, or both.

Problem

Laparoscopy is a hybrid surgical approach that shares characteristics of both minor and major surgery.

To patients, laparoscopic procedures often seem to be minor surgery because of the small incisions, relatively less postoperative pain, and short convalescent period.

When a laparoscopic procedure involves minimal intra-abdominal surgery, both postoperative discomfort and the risk of complications may more closely resemble a minor procedure than a major procedure.

At its essence, laparoscopy remains an intra-abdominal procedure; therefore, it shares all intraoperative and postoperative risks of laparotomy, including infection and injury to adjacent intra-abdominal structures.

When major intra-abdominal procedures are performed laparoscopically, the resultant postoperative pain and morbidity are still significant.

However, because a large abdominal incision is unnecessary, the postoperative pain and morbidity are always less than similar major surgery performed by laparotomy.

Laparoscopic procedures have unique risks, which are related to methods used for the placement of abdominal wall ports, the pneumoperitoneum required for laparoscopy and use of energy within the abdominal cavity.

These risks include injury to bowel, bladder, or major blood vessels and intravascular insufflation.

In addition, increased intra-abdominal pressures with laparoscopy increase anesthesia-related risks such as aspiration and increased difficulty ventilating the patient.

Although the risk of blood loss is relatively low for most procedures, potentially massive blood loss may occur and is complicated by the fact that control of blood loss may be delayed by the time taken to perform an emergency laparotomy.

HYSTEROSCOPY

EVOLUTION OF HYSTEROSCOPY

Hysteroscopy involves the passage of a small diameter telescope either flexible or rigid, through the cervix to directly inspect the uterine cavity.

The introduction of hysteroscopy in gynecologic practice revolutionized the diagnosis and treatment of intrauterine disease.

New methodologic and technologic developments have made diagnostic and operative hysteroscopy much more efficient, cost effective, safe, and useful.

The development of hysteroscopy is rooted in the work of Pantaleoni, who first reported uterine endoscopy in 1869.

However, at that time, instrumentation was elementary, and expansion of the uterine cavity was insufficient.

In 1925, Rubin first used CO_2 to distend the uterus. Around the same time, Gauss was experimenting with the use of fluids to achieve uterine expansion.

Hysteroscopy did not become popular until the 1970s, when technology afforded more practical and usable instruments than before.

The use of liquid distention media became routine by the 1980s, and many new hysteroscopic procedures, including endometrial ablation, were developed.

Initially used by urologists for transurethral resection of the prostate, the resectoscope was modified for hysteroscopic procedures, allowing for resection of intrauterine pathology with monopolar cautery.

By the mid-1980s, hysteroscopic procedures had nearly replaced D&C for diagnosing intrauterine pathology.

Thus, hysteroscopy is apparently the oldest endoscopic procedure described in medical literature.

In today's field of obstetrics and gynecology, hysteroscopy has become a cornerstone in evaluating and treating infertile women and those with functional or anatomical uterine anomalies.

Minimally invasive surgery has experienced a boom over the last 20 years, resulting in a wide expansion of techniques and indications for diagnostic as well as operative hysteroscopy. In the field of diagnostic hysteroscopy, numerous innovations have entered the clinical routine, among them small-diameter rigid and flexible hysteroscopes.

Over the past few decades, refinements in optic and fiberoptic technology and inventions of new surgical accessories have dramatically improved visual resolution and surgical techniques in hysteroscopy.

Many hysteroscopic procedures have replaced old, invasive techniques. Now, as instruments become smaller than before, office hysteroscopy is replacing operating-room procedures.

One of the most recent hysteroscopic procedures approved by the US Food and Drug Administration (FDA) is female sterilization (Essure, Conceptus, Incorporated, Mountain View, Calif), which can be performed in the gynecologist's office. Novel instruments and techniques continue to emerge, and the prospects for improvement seem unlimited.

INDICATIONS OF HYSTEROSCOPY

Hysteroscopy has become, in the last years, a great work-up method in gynecology, and it is considered the gold standard approach to intrauterine pathologies.

The remarkable progress in technological development associated with an improvement in medical training and ability with the relative simplicity of the technique have made hysteroscopy a simple, secure and highly accurate method to access the cervical canal, uterine cavity and tubal ostium, and widen the indications for hysteroscopy.

It is in the field of improved diagnosis that hysteroscopy has made the most significant progress, mainly because the ability to use fine diameter instruments makes it feasible to avoid both anaesthesia and cervical dilatation.

Today diagnostic hysteroscopy can be considered the optimal method of assessing all cases where visualizing the cervical canal, uterine cavity and tubal ostea will improve diagnostic accuracy and guide therapeutic management through an outpatient setting with minimum discomfort to women.

During reproductive life, the appearance of the endometrium varies according to the menstrual cycle and the patient's hormonal status.

Following menstruation and until the 10th day of the cycle, the endometrium is pale, the surface is smooth, and the thickness measured by making a crease with the optic on the posterior wall will be 3 to 4mm.

From the 11th to 13th day, the endometrium is more congested, redder in color and with a thickness of 6 mm; the glandular orifices are more visible.

During the ovulatory phase and for further 48 to 72 hours, the endometrium once again becomes pale, very thick (7 to 8 mm); reflects light and because of the edema is much more succulent.

The glands are only slightly exposed in relief and there is a serous intracavitary fluid. Carbon dioxide can easily form bubbles in this fluid.

In the secretory phase, the edematous aspect will disappear by about the 3rd postovulatory day and with it the intracavitary fluid will be dispersed.

The cavity distends more easily and the endometrium appears more pink, lightly folded, and at a magnification x20 times, the glands stand out in relief on the surface, taking on a pseudocystic appearance, the capillary vessels are more apparent surrounding the glandular orifices, these vessels will take a spiral aspect immediately before the menstruation.

Infertility

During the last few years, diagnostic hysteroscopy has become a valuable tool in the evaluation and treatment of infertility and recurrent pregnancy loss.

Due to the high incidence of uterine cavity pathologies and improvement of reproductive outcome after surgical correction, it is significant to evaluate the uterine cavity accurately in infertile patients.

Indications of hysteroscopy for infertility include; abnormal hysterogram, abnormal uterine bleeding, suspected intrauterine pathology, uterine anomalies, unexplained infertility, pregnancy wastage, planned intrauterine surgery, polyps, submucous leiomyomas, uterine septa, intrauterine adhesions, misplaced or embedded foreign bodies and tubal cannulation.

It has been frequently advised to perform hysteroscopy as a routine procedure prior to IVF/ICSI treatment.

Additional pathology which can interfere with embryo implantation and development are uterine malformations, particularly a septate uterus, although uterine malformations are usually associated with pregnancy wastage, not infertility.

Hysteroscopy and laparoscopy allow precise classification and consequently appropriate treatment of uterine malformations.

When facing the problem of recurrent abortion, visualization of the uterine cavity becomes indispensable for a correct diagnosis, and forms the basis for an appropriate therapy.

Intracavitary lesions are implicated as causes of infertility, and their removal may increase fertility.

In general, studies have suggested that hysteroscopic removal of lesions <2 cm does not adversely affect an IVF cycle.

The effect of myomas on reproduction is not definitive but it is generally accepted that fibroids causing distortion of the endometrial cavity may adversely influence fertility.

Location, size of myomas, and coexisting fertility diagnoses are believed to be major considerations when determining management options.

Debate also exists in regard to management of small myomas with minimal uterine cavity distortion.

For patients with recurrent miscarriage and intracavitary fibroids, surgery increases rates of viable pregnancy outcomes.

Myomas may adversely affect outcomes for women undergoing IVF but there again remains no definitive consensus on management of fibroids prior to an IVF attempt.

The frequency of unsuspected intrauterine pathology has been reported to be 40% by routine hysteroscopy.

The types and frequencies of the subtle pathologies were as follows: endometrial polyps -- 65%, endometrial hyperplasia -- 17%, endometrial hypotrophia -- 13%, and other endometritis, adhesion -- 5%.

Congenital Uterine Anomalies

Approximately 1-2% of all women, 4% of infertile women, and 10-15% of patients with recurrent miscarriage have Müllerian anomalies.

These anomalies range from didelphys to Müllerian agenesis.

Uterine septum and in utero DES exposure are more likely to be associated with miscarriage than is uterus didelphys.

Patients with a bicornuate uterus have a >50% live birth rate compared with those with a uterine septum, who have a <30% live birth rate.

Patients with in utero DES exposure are likely to have a T-shaped uterus with corneal restriction bands, pretubal bulges, lower-uterine-segment dilation, and a small and irregular cavity with borders resembling adhesions.

Hysteroscopy can be used to confirm but not always to treat these findings.

Septate uterus is the most common structural uterine anomaly, accounting for 35% of anomalies, and is associated with the highest incidence of reproductive failure.

The diagnosis of septate uterus is made after excluding the diagnosis of a bicornuate uterus.

Once 2 hemicavities are visualized on imaging, the uterine fundus must be evaluated by laparoscopy.

Evidence of fundal indentation is an indication of bicornuate uterus, whereas, a smooth fundus is present with uterine septum.

Division of a uterine septum has historically been performed by laparotomy but is now most commonly performed via a hysteroscopic approach.

Edstrom reported the first hysteroscopic resection of a septum, and Bret and Guillet were the first to recommend incising versus excising the septum.

Hysteroscopic metroplasty in women with septate uterus significantly improves reproductive outcomes.

Surgical complications are fewer with the hysteroscopic approach than with other procedures, such as Jones, Strassman, or Tompkins metroplasty.

Of patients undergoing hysteroscopic resection for Müllerian anomalies, 20% have dysmenorrhea after surgery compared with 50% after abdominal procedures.

Rates of term-pregnancy outcomes after hysteroscopic resection are equivalent to those of abdominal metroplasty for uterine septum, and live birth rates after treatment are as high as 80%.

Significant improvements are seen in pregnancy outcomes following hysteroscopic metroplasty in women with recurrent miscarriage.

Pregnancy rates have been estimated to increase to approximately 80% after hysteroscopic correction with a significant decrease in miscarriage rates.

Although, a septate uterus is not a cause for infertility, the literature suggests women with a septate uterus and otherwise unexplained infertility may benefit from metroplasty, but to a more modest extent.

Metroplasty should also be considered for women who plan to undergo IVF.

Polyps and Fibroids

Endometrial polyps and fibroids are well known to cause irregular vaginal bleeding.

Fibroids are the most common solid pelvic tumor in women, found in 20% of women older than 35 years.

Menorrhagia due to symptomatic submucosal fibroids is the most common indication for surgical intervention.

Other indications include infertility, dysmenorrhea, and pelvic pain.

Polyps and submucosal fibroids can be definitively diagnosed and effectively treated with hysteroscopy.

Diagnosis of endometrial polyps via hysteroscopy is 94% sensitive and 92% specific.

For submucosal myomas, diagnostic hysteroscopy is 87% sensitive and 95% specific.

Initial hysteroscopy is estimated to successfully remove fibroids in 85-95% of cases, with additional surgery required in approximately 5-15%.

Recurrence of symptoms after hysteroscopic myomectomy is most common with large uteri and numerous and deep fibroids.

The advantages of hysteroscopic resection are numerous and include treating irregular bleeding and obtaining tissue diagnosis; for myomectomy, benefits include avoiding laparotomy, uterine incision, and hospital stay.

If a fibroid is predominantly submucosal, complete resection is possible.

A 2-step procedure is sometimes needed to resect a fibroid that is partially intramural or large.

In patients desiring fertility, hysteroscopic myomectomy is a reasonable option and minimal cauterization should be used to decrease damage to otherwise healthy endometrium.

Intrauterine Adhesions

Asherman syndrome was identified in 1948 as uterine synechiae.

These IUAs are often associated with amenorrhea or infertility.

The prevalence rate of IUAs in the general population is 1.5%, with adhesions noted in up to 30% of women undergoing hysteroscopy following 3 or more spontaneous abortions treated with D&C.

Hysteroscopy is the gold standard used to diagnose and treat these adhesions.

Filmy adhesions are often lysed by distention alone, whereas the dense adhesions often require cutting or excision with blunt, sharp, electrocautery, or laser techniques.

If the patient's symptoms include abnormal bleeding, hysteroscopic treatment results in an 88-98% return to normal menstrual cycles.

If no other infertility issues are present, 79% of treated patients have normal pregnancies i.e, 75% of those with mild disease but only 31% with severe adhesions.

Reformation of adhesions may have a significant impact on the conception rate after hysteroscopic adhesiolysis.

Conception rates in women with recurrence of adhesions after initial hysteroscopic adhesiolysis have been found to be significantly lower than in women with demonstration of a normal uterine cavity on second look hysteroscopy.

Of consideration, hysteroscopic treatment may also increase the risk of abnormal placentation (eg, accreta, percreta, increta, previa).

Proximal Tubal Obstruction

This diagnosis is difficult to make and is most often suggested by HSG.

It may be due to infection, intraluminal debris, salpingitis isthmica nodosum, endometriosis, or may simply be due to spasm.

In theory, repair of proximal disease and removal of scar tissue is beneficial, and cannulation of the tubes can be performed at the same time.

Tubal perforation is rare but could lead to further tubal pathology.

Reocclusion occurs in approximately one third of cases.

Up to 85% of occlusions can be treated with cannulation.

HYSTEROSCOPY: Indications

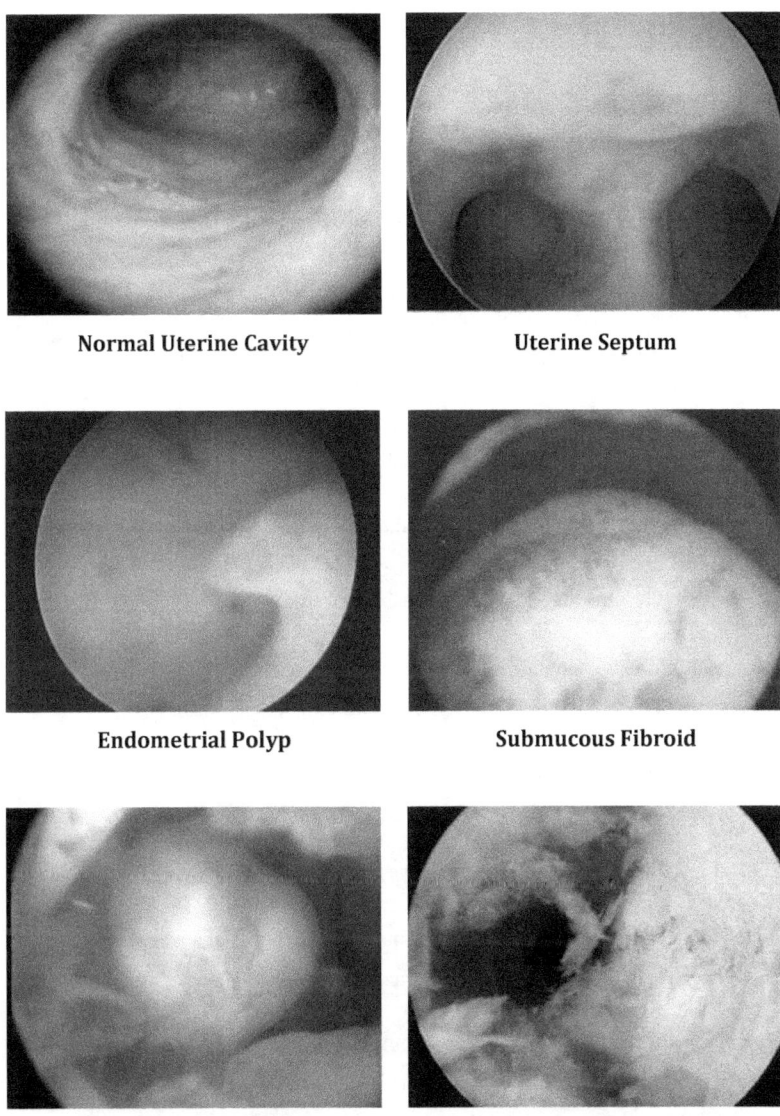

Normal Uterine Cavity — Uterine Septum

Endometrial Polyp — Submucous Fibroid

Submucous Fibroid Polyp — Intrauterine Adhesions

Hysteroscopy: Indications

EQUIPMENT OF HYSTEROSCOPY

The basic equipment used to perform diagnostic hysteroscopy includes the hysteroscope, light source, and distention media.

Modern systems use a digital camera that attaches to the eyepiece and transmits images to a visual monitoring screen.

Diagnostic hysteroscopes are available in different sizes: the choice of a particular type can affect pain tolerance, image quality, and intraoperative surgical options.

The hysteroscope usually includes the telescope and the sheath that encases it; newer diagnostic models, however, may lack the sheath.

Outer sheaths have accessory channels that enable the inflow and outflow of the distention media.

When applicable, the sheath and a separate connecting bridge also have ports to insert operative and manipulating instruments, the 2 instrument dimensions of great consequence are the outer diameter (OD) and working length (WL).

The OD indicates the width of the barrel including the sheath.

For diagnostic hysteroscopes that do not use a sheath, the OD refers only to the width of the optic barrel.

Modern hysteroscopes range from 2.7-10 mm; the OD of a diagnostic scope typically ranges from 2.7-5.0 mm, while the OD of an operative sheath ranges from 5-10 mm.

Rigid scopes with an OD exceeding 5.0 mm usually require some degree of cervical dilation, while use of a narrow caliber (or flexible) hysteroscope usually requires no cervical dilation.

The WL measures the distance between the distal lens to the proximal eyepiece and ranges from 160-302 mm.

Longer WLs permit the surgeon to operate farther from the vagina and may be of importance in the morbidly obese patient.

The 3 parts of the hysteroscope (excluding the sheath) are the lens, the barrel, and the eyepiece.

The depth of field on the scope is usually between 2-3 cm, and magnification can reach up to 35X with certain liquid distention media and lens positioning.

Hysteroscopes are available in a variety of viewing angles: 0°, 12°, 15°, 25°, 30°, and 70°.

Zero degree scopes provide a wide-angled view in-line with the barrel.

Angled scopes allow for clear views of the periphery without requiring excessive operator movement and are often helpful to visualize the tubal ostia.

Cameras that attach to the eyepiece are frequently used to transmit images to a video monitor.

Electronic displays allow the operating room personnel to watch the procedure and are convenient for intraoperative teaching.

These systems are also capable of electronically documenting the procedure with still images and video clips for future reference.

Light Source

Satisfactory sources of "cold" light using halogen or xenon lamps have been available for several years.

A xenon light source with a liquid cable is considered the superior option.

Distention Media

The uterine cavity is a potential space; hysteroscopic examination requires the cavity be distended with either gas or liquid.

The use of hysteroscopic monopolar or bipolar energy limits the choice of distention media.

Because diagnostic hysteroscopy typically does not require the use of an electrical energy source, many options are available for the patient and surgeon.

Gas Distension Media

The only gas used in diagnostic hysteroscopy is CO_2.

Carbon dioxide is a safe distension media when used at pressures below the mean arterial pressure (MAP) of approximately 100 mmHg and flow rates less than 100 ml per min.

The advantages of CO_2 include high solubility in blood, high image clarity, and ubiquity in all operating rooms equipped for laparoscopy.

Its use for hysteroscopy is limited to diagnostic cases and has significant disadvantages: the combination of intrauterine blood and CO_2 creates bubbles that can dramatically reduce the viewable area and limit the diagnostic survey.

The use of CO_2 in hysteroscopy also requires the use of a hysteron-insufflator.

Laparoscopic insufflation devices are absolutely contraindicated because they cannot provide low rates of flow (30-100 ml per min) and safely limit the intrauterine pressure to less than 100 mmHg.

Unintentional use of laparoscopic insufflators can cause CO_2 embolisms that have led to cardiac arrhythmias and death.

Fluid Distension Media

The main advantage of fluid over gas is its ability to flush blood and tissue out of the viewing field.

Fluid media can be functionally categorized into 2 groups: electrolyte and non-electrolyte.

The choice of media should take into consideration the patient co-morbidities and the possibility of adding an operative component to the diagnostic procedure.

Electrolyte-containing solutions include normal saline (NS) and lactated Ringer's solution (LR).

Both are low viscosity fluids that are capable of conducting electric current.

Neither can be used in procedures requiring monopolar energy.

Advantages of electrolyte solutions include compatibility with mechanical, laser, or bipolar energy sources and decreased concern for electrolyte imbalance from fluid extra-vasation.

Disadvantages of electrolyte solutions include their miscibility with blood and their electrical conductivity.

Nonelectrolyte solutions include 1.5% glycine, 3% sorbitol, 5% mannitol, and 5% dextrose.

With the exception of isotonic 5% mannitol, these low-viscosity solutions are hypotonic and nonconductive.

Unlike NS and LR, they are all compatible with monopolar energy systems.

The hypotonicity of these solutions imparts a risk of hyponatremia when absorbed in large volumes.

Fluid deficits above 1500 ml or serum sodium of less than 125 should prompt the immediate termination of the procedure and serial monitoring of postoperative blood chemistries.

Glycine is metabolized to ammonia and should not be used in patients with significant hepatic dysfunction.

Sorbitol is quickly metabolized into fructose and glucose and should be avoided in patients with impaired glucose tolerance.

Evidence has suggested that 5% mannitol may be the safest of all nonelectrolyte solutions given its ability to remain in the extracellular compartment and maintain serum osmolarity in the setting of concurrent hyponatremia.

High-viscosity fluids are used in hysteroscopy to limit image distortion due to intrauterine bleeding.

Currently, the only high-viscosity fluid option is Dextran 70; Dextran 70 is void of electrolytes and is therefore nonconductive.

Simplicity of use and excellent light transmission are among the advantages of Dextran 70.

The advantages of its high viscosity are that it does not escape easily through the fallopian tubes or cervix and so maintains uterine distension and that it does not mix with blood.

The disadvantages are that it may be difficult to infuse through the hysteroscope and that the instruments must be washed immediately in warm water to prevent crystallization of the fluid and blockage of stop-cocks.

There have also been occasional reports of allergic reactions and anaphylaxis, fluid overload, disseminated intravascular coagulopathy.

For every 100 ml absorbed, the plasma volume can expand an additional 860 ml.

Because intrauterine Dextran 70 absorption can occur after administration of volumes as low as 50-100 ml, actively monitoring fluid deficit and immediately terminating the procedure if the deficit reaches 500 ml is important.

Care must be taken to wash the devices in hot water immediately after the surgery to prevent damage to the instrument by hardened Dextran.

Intraoperative fluid management is an important aspect of hysteroscopy; the use of an automated fluid management system is recommended.

These systems provide real-time information about the fluid deficit and can also actively manage intrauterine pressures.

A member of the operating room personnel should be designated to call out the deficit when it reaches 500 ml and every additional 100 ml.

With the exception of Dextran 70, the surgeon should plan for completion of the case if the fluid deficit reaches 750 ml.

The procedure should be immediately terminated if deficits reach 1500 ml for nonelectrolyte solutions or 2500 ml for isotonic solutions like NS or LR.

If high volume deficits are suspected, electrolytes should be measured and diuretics given as indicated.

Of note, hysteroscopic systems with ports for both inflow and outflow are superior in recording accurate fluid levels and decrease the amount of fluid left unaccounted on the table, drapes, and floor.

If automated systems are unavailable, the distention fluid media can be administered and measured manually.

Optical Systems

Optical systems are either rigid or flexible.

The main technical difference between the two systems is being the mode of image transmission.

The flexible hysteroscope is most commonly used for office hysteroscopy and has recently gained popularity; it is notable for its flexibility, with a tip that deflects over a range of 120-160.

Its most appropriate use is to accommodate the irregularly shaped uterus and to navigate around intrauterine lesions.

It is also used for diagnostic and operative procedures.

During insertion, the flexible contour accommodates to the cervix more easily than does a rigid scope of a similarly small diameter.

The view was initially described as having a ground-glass quality, which was markedly less desirable than the view obtained with rigid scopes.

New, digitally enhanced scopes now offer similar image quality to a rigid hysteroscope lens.

Rigid hysteroscopes are the most commonly used instruments.

Their wide range of diameters allows for in-office and complex operating-room procedures.

Of the narrow options (3- 5 mm in diameter), the 4-mm scope offers the sharpest and clearest view.

It accommodates surgical instruments but is small enough to require minimal cervical dilation.

In addition, patients tolerate this instrument well with only paracervical block anesthesia.

Rigid scopes larger than 5 mm in diameter (commonly 8-10 mm) require increased cervical dilation for insertion.

Therefore, they are most frequently used in the operating room with IV sedation or general anesthesia.

Large instruments include an outer sheath to introduce and remove media and to provide ports to accommodate large and varied surgical instruments.

Three types of rigid lens systems are in use: Hopkins, Lumina and Olympus.

Optical systems have angles of vision ranging from 0 to 30 degrees, the latter being the most popular.

Their external diameter can be as little as 1.2 mm.

This diameter makes the device less durable but does not reduce visibility.

An instrument 4 to 5 mm in diameter is considered preferable for routine use because it still permits endoscopic examination without anesthesia or cervical dilatation.

Hamou's microhysteroscope has two advantages over other systems for diagnostic hysteroscopy: a fine diameter (5mm) essential for performing the examination in the outpatient clinic and a system of lenses controlled by a push button switch which offers 4 magnifications: x1, x20, x60 and x150.

Lower magnifications (x1 and x20) are used to obtain a panoramic view of the uterine cavity.

This is similar to the view obtained with a colposcope for the ecto-cervix and comparable to the traditional hysteroscope for the examination of the cervical canal and uterine cavity.

Higher magnifications of x60 and x150) require contact vision after vital staining of the area and show the structure and arrangement of the surface cellular layers.

Changing the magnification is easy and carried out by simply pressing a push-button switch on the side of the device during the course of the examination.

Specially designed for the office use, the new generation of small diameter hysteroscopes (3.5 mm) in combination with an atraumatic insertion technique allows success rates of almost 98% for diagnostic hysteroscopy; therefore, hysteroscopy is now generally acknowledged as the "gold standard" investigation of the uterine cavity.

The narrow diameter of the hysteroscope and its manouverability permit easy and relatively painless exploration of both the cervical canal and uterine cavity.

The continuous insufflation of CO_2 creates the desired dilatation of the cervical canal as well as of the uterine cavity.

HYSTEROSCOPY: Equipment

Distension with a continuous flow of liquid requires a double sheath for infusion and aspiration.

Continuous liquid flow is indicated in patients with bleeding because always it can maintain a clear vision.

Rigid versus Flexible Hysteroscopy

Hysteroscopes can be classified into rigid and flexible (or semi-rigid) types.

Rigid hysteroscopes require some assembly.

Most designs require that the telescope be inserted into a sheath that is then attached to a bridge.

Bridges for a diagnostic scope may only have a single inflow port.

Operative bridges typically have 2 media ports with additional ports for instruments.

Dual media ports for inflow and outflow can produce a steady laminar flow to improve image clarity during procedures in which blood can obscure the field of view.

A growing number of very narrow, flexible hysteroscopes that produce less pain and are more suitable for outpatient applications are available.

Flexible scopes are available in diagnostic and operative models and can have an OD as small as 2.7 mm.

In a trial randomizing 144 women to either flexible or rigid diagnostic hysteroscopy, women in the rigid group experienced significantly more pain than those in the flexible group.

Physicians, however, reported better optical quality with the rigid scope when compared with the flexible scope.

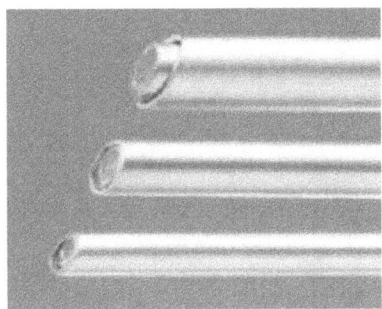 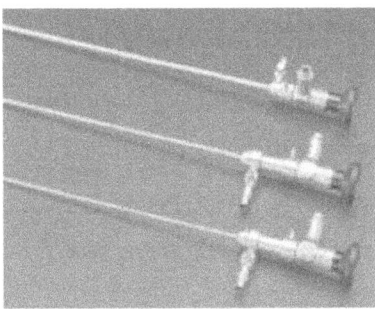

Diagnostic Hysteroscope

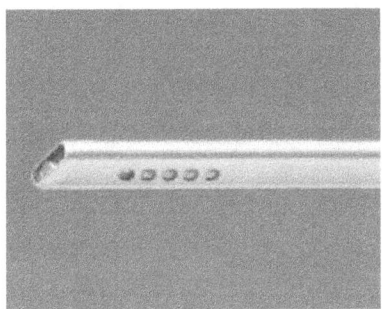 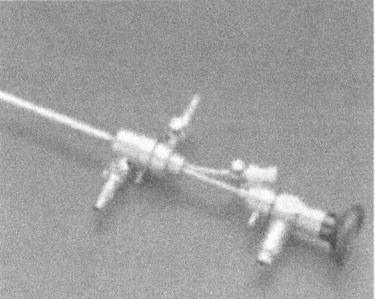

Operative Hysteroscope

Hysteroscopy: Equipment

RELEVANT ANATOMY

For any hysteroscopic procedure, the surgeon must understand the thickness of the uterine wall.

This knowledge allows the surgeon to manipulate the surgery on the basis of the area of the uterus where he is operating.

Uterine Wall Thickness

Site \ Thickness	Minimum (mm)	Maximum (mm)	Mean (mm)
– Anterior wall	17	25	22.5
– Posterior wall	15	25	21
– Fundus	15	22	19.5
– Isthmus	8	12	10
– Corpus	4	7	5.5

TECHNIQUE OF HYSTEROSCOPY

The most important challenge for the office approach is to reduce patient discomfort to a minimum.

This should not be underestimated since many patients still prefer the inpatient approach believing that it will be pain free.

Pain is the main limiting factor to the outpatient procedure and one of the causes of impaired accuracy of the exam, sometimes leading to unsatisfactory results.

So several alternatives have been proposed for pain reduction during office diagnostic hysteroscopy, but the results are still inconclusive.

Over the last years, major technical improvements, such as the use of saline as distension medium, the availability of high-resolution mini-endoscopes and the atraumatic insertion of the instruments, have led to the development of the mini-hysteroscopy.

This technique avoids most traumatic uterine maneuvers leading to a less painful and better tolerated examination and has increased the feasibility and acceptability of the office diagnostic hysteroscopy.

Therefore, it is now recommended as a first line diagnostic tool for the evaluation of abnormal uterine bleeding (AUB), and infertility, and also for operative purposes.

The advantages of the mini-hysteroscopy have been reported in many studies.

It seems logical to schedule the hysteroscopies during the proliferative phase in infertile patients to avoid the potential risk of carrying out it in the presence of an early pregnancy if it is performing in the second half of the menstrual cycle.

Examinations during the secretory phase should be avoided to allow for optimal views of the cavity since secretory endometrium can mimic intrauterine pathology.

The patient should be examined and a speculum introduced.

A tenaculum is placed on the anterior lip of the cervix for traction.

At this time local anesthesia can be used, if appropriate, by injecting a few ml of carbocaine 2% into the cervix.

Vaginal misoprostol prior to diagnostic hysteroscopy reduces cervical resistance in nonpregnant women.

The hysteroscope is gently introduced in the cervical canal and advanced under visual control into the uterine cavity.

The ecto-cervix and vaginal fornix, cervical canal and uterine cavity may be explored.

During examination of the ectocervix low magnification (x1, x20) provides results that are comparable with those obtained by colposcopy, although traditional colposcopy presents clear advantages because the colposcope allows a more accurate observation of fine details which are so crucial in cervical pathology.

The field of vision of the colposcope is wider and is not deformed by the 30 degree angle view afforded by the hysteroscope.

Some advocate vaginoscopic "no-touch" hysteroscopy as a more painless technique.

Such an approach forgoes the speculum and tenaculum and begins with vaginal and cervical disinfection followed by the intravaginal introduction of a rigid hysteroscope.

The external cervical os is identified using the instrument light, and the examination is conducted as usual.

If a liquid distention media is used, intrauterine placement and orientation can be confirmed by visualizing bubbles at 12 o'clock.

Once the distal tip of the hysteroscope is just inside the uterine cavity, allow the media to expand the intrauterine space.

Adjustments to the rates of media inflow and outflow are done to expand the cavity, optimize image quality, and create smooth laminar flow.

The intrauterine space is then ready for systematic inspection.

The first evaluation should be a panoramic view of the intrauterine cavity.

Next, careful inspection of the following areas should be done: lateral uterine walls, superior uterine cavity, and anterior and posterior uterine walls.

Gentle movement of the hysteroscope is imperative.

Excessive trauma to the endometrial surface causes bleeding that obscures the view, increases systemic fluid absorption, and risks perforation.

Any pathology should be inspected and documented.

If hysteroscopy is being performed to evaluate endometrial polyps or other intrauterine pathology, tissue samples can be obtained with hysteroscopic forceps followed by D&C after hysteroscopy.

When the diagnostic survey is complete, the hysteroscope is slowly withdrawn.

Careful inspection during removal provides one final chance to inspect the endocervical canal.

A complete diagnostic hysteroscopy should take approximately 10-15 minutes.

Recovery after diagnostic hysteroscopy is prompt.

If no anesthesia is used, patients can return to their usual diet and activities later that operative day.

Pharmacologic Endometrial Preparation

Endometrial preparation is typically performed prior to operative hysteroscopy but may be necessary prior to diagnostic hysteroscopy, especially in anovulatory patients.

Pharmacologic thinning of the endometrium can be done with a course of progestins, oral contraceptives, danazol, or GnRH agonists.

Use of a Tenaculum

Placement of a tenaculum on the anterior cervix is often the first cause of pain during a diagnostic hysteroscopy.

With the availability of small diameter flexible scopes, most diagnostic procedures can be performed without a tenaculum.

In the event that a tenaculum is needed, pain can be decreased with a topical anesthetic or by infiltrating the area of placement with local anesthetic using a 22-gauge to 25-gauge spinal needle.

Nonsteroidal Anti-Inflammatory Drugs

The use of oral or intravenous analgesics in the preoperative period is common.

Nonsteroidal anti-inflammatory drugs (NSAID) have been shown to reduce only postoperative pain with minimal effect on intraoperative pain and may be a good choice for some patients.

Anaesthesia and Analgesia

Severe pain and patient anxiety are among the most common causes of surgical failure.

Many anesthetic options are available to patients undergoing hysteroscopy.

For hysteroscopes of larger diameter, injectable local anesthetic combined with preoperative vaginal misoprostol is usually sufficient.

Occasionally, regional anesthesia, monitored anesthesia care (MAC), or general anesthesia may be indicated for more extensive procedures or for patients who have lower pain tolerance and/or anxiety.

Many practitioners favor the use of topical anesthesia, although studies have shown mixed efficacy.

Aerosolized preparations of lidocaine may decrease cervical pain from tenaculum placement but do not decrease uterine sensation.

Topical anesthetics typically do not provide long-lasting relief but may be sufficient for the nonanesthetized patient.

Paracervical Block

A paracervical block can decrease the pain of tenaculum placement, cervical dilation, and hysteroscope insertion through the cervix.

However, paracervical anesthesia has less effect on the pain of uterine distension.

One must balance the expected pain of the hysteroscopic procedure with the pain and potential side-effects of the paracervical block, which include bradycardia and hypotension.

For these reasons, many providers choose to forgo this step, especially for brief diagnostic procedures.

Common anesthetic agents are 1% lidocaine, mepivacaine, prilocaine, ropivacaine, bupivacaine, and etidocaine. Of these, bupivacaine and etidocaine have longer durations and can last upwards of 2-3 hours.

In most cases, 10 ml of bupivacaine 0.25%, mepivacaine 1%, or lidocaine 1-2% is an adequate volume for paracervical anesthesia.

Misoprostol

Patients with cervical stenosis may require some cervical dilation for diagnostic hysteroscopy, especially after menopause.

Misoprostol, a synthetic prostaglandin E_1 analogue, may be administered orally or vaginally for cervical ripening to improve the likelihood of successful cervical dilation and decrease intraoperative pain with few adverse events.

HYSTEROSCOPY: Technique

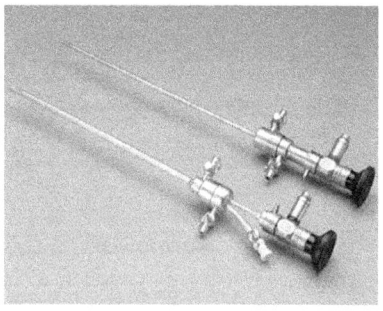 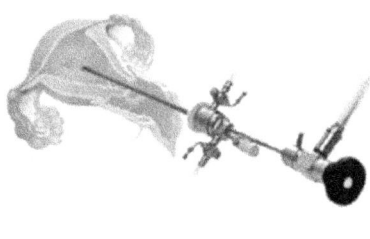

Rigid Hysteroscope

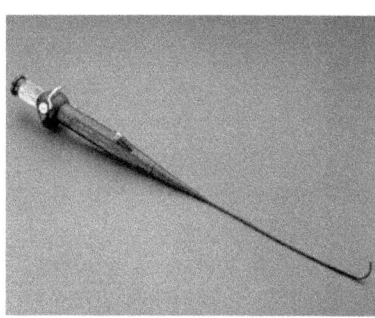 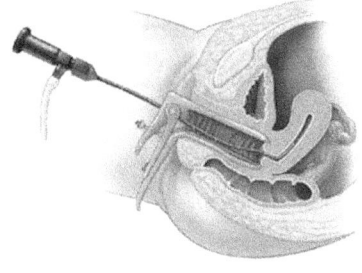

Flexible Hysteroscope

Hysteroscopy: Technique

COMPLICATIONS OF HYSTEROSCOPY

Diagnostic hysteroscopy is a safe procedure with good patient acceptability and minimal pain.

Complications which may result from anesthesia, positioning the patient or the distension media are uterine perforation, haemorrhage and delayed complications which are infection, adhesion formation and failure of resolution of the presenting symptoms.

The outpatient hysteroscopy failure rate is less than half (2%) with the mini-hysteroscope compared with the traditional 5 mm hysteroscope (5%).

Risk of vasovagal syndrome is higher with the use of a rigid hysteroscope and CO_2, regardless of the indication for hysteroscopy or the parity and menopausal status of the patient.

The prevalence of vagal reaction depends on the ability of the endoscopist and on the diameter of the scope.

Regarding pain; the literature suggests that outpatient hysteroscopy without any form of analgesia or anaesthesia is a welltolerated procedure with a high success rate.

Indeed, pain experienced during the procedure can occur even if local anaesthesia is used.

Thus, pain continues to represent the main limiting factor to a large scale use of office hysteroscopy.

To minimize patient's discomfort and maximize the chance of success of theprocedure and its widespread use, a new technique based on the employment of small-diameter rigid and flexible hysteroscopes and an atraumatic insertion technique (vaginoscopic approach) has been developed.

HYSTEROSCOPY: Complications

This technique has permitted complete elimination of any kind of premedication, analgesia or anaesthesia, making the procedure faster and complication-free.

The most frequent complications seen during hysteroscopy are the result of over distension of the uterine cavity.

The uterus can be adequately distended with a pressure of 60 to 80 mmHg of CO_2.

Automatic "hysteroflators" keep of CO_2 flow under 80 ml/min and maintain an intrauterine pressure less than 100 mm Hg and make the procedure very safe.

Bleeding during or after surgery is the second most common complication of hysteroscopy (0.25%); where myomectomy is the procedure with the highest complication rate (23%).

Data suggest improvements in blood loss and preprocedural hematocrit levels when patients are pretreated with GnRH agonists or oral contraceptives.

Distention media themselves may yield enough pressure to cause hemostasis during a procedure.

In addition, the coagulating effects of surgical instruments can aid in controlling bleeding during surgery.

Mild bleeding is typically self-limited and generally does not require intervention.

If brisk bleeding occurs, electrocautery may be used to coagulate small vessels.

If these conservative approaches fail to control heavy bleeding or if there is bleeding from larger vessels, a Foley catheter or intrauterine balloon can be inserted into the cavity and inflated to tamponade the hemorrhage.

Complications can also occur when using Dextran 70 "Hyskon".

They include pulmonary edema, and coagulopathy consequent to intravasation, the proposed mechanisms are fluid overload, toxic effects of Dextran 70 on the pulmonary capillaries, and/or probable anticoagulant effects.

Fluid overload is a rare complication especially in diagnostic hysteroscopy, it is more common in surgical myomectomy and endometrial ablation but rare in polypectomy.

Risk factors for clinically significant intravasation of fluid include prolonged operative procedures, use of large volumes of low viscosity media, resection of fibroids or myometrial trauma that results in open uterine venous channels or unidentified perforations.

One of the ways found to control the amount of liquid absorbed by the patient is the assessment of the difference between the amount of medium that is being infused during the procedure and the amount that is being absorbed.

This deficit should not exceed 1500 ml to avoid fluid overload.

Liquid intravasation can cause clinically significant overload in long surgical procedures; maximal absorption should not exceed 500 ml.

This type of overload does not respond to diuretic treatment because the kidneys poorly excrete Dextran 70.

This problem may be compounded by not decreasing the rate of IV fluid administration to compensate for the hysteroscopic absorption of distension media.

Additionally, the uptake of relatively small volumes of Dextran 70 can lead to significant intravascular volume expansion because of the fluid's osmotic properties.

The initial clinical symptoms of excessive absorption of distension medium are nausea, vomiting, headache, and motor agitation.

If not promptly and adequately treated, thepatient may develop pulmonary and cerebral edema and even death.

Therefore it is of utmost importance that both the surgical team and anesthetic team are constantly communicating, because if the patient begins to manifest such symptoms the procedure should be interrupted immediately, and appropriate treatment started, and monitoring of the patient intensified.

Anaphylaxis is another complication of Dextran 70, with frequencies of 1 case per 1500-300,000 patients.

Treatment of anaphylaxis includes diphenhydramine, epinephrine, steroids, and possible fluid and ventilatory support. Disseminated intravascular coagulopathy and adult respiratory distress syndrome are life threatening complications of hysteroscopy.

Uterine perforation is one of the complications occurred during hysteroscopy.

The incidence of perforation is about 0.7-3%.

It usually occurs in difficult cases during dilatation of the cervix or during adhesiolysis followed by myomectomy and septum resection.

Risk factors for perforation include cervical stenosis, severe uterine anteflexion or retroflexion, infection, myomas of lower uterine segments, and synechiae.

Perforation occurs more frequently at the level of the fundus without significant bleeding.

When perforation occurs laparoscopy should be performed and antibiotics and oxytocin administered for at least two days.

Because of excellent drainage, the risk for infection with office hysteroscopy is exceedingly low (0.1%-2.8%).

An incidence of 0.2% of infection in over 4000 diagnostic hysteroscopies has been reported.

If a patient has a preoperative infection or a significant history of PID, treatment before surgery is recommended, but prophylactic antibiotics do not reduce the risk of infection after surgery.

CONTRAINDICATIONS OF HYSTEROSCOPY

Pregnancy in the premenopausal patient should always be excluded with serum or urine B-hCG testing prior to surgery.

Hysteroscopy should not be performed in the setting of cervical or endometrial cancer.

The technique does not have absolute contraindications but, in general, it is not indicated in acute PID, mucopurulent cervicitis, after recent uterine perforation and when risks and benefits should be considered.

Treatment of pelvic infections is mandatory prior to hysteroscopy to decrease the chance of gynecologic infections that can lead to pelvic pain, tubal factor infertility, and even death.

In general, hysteroscopy is avoided in patients with; active cervical or uterine infection, a large uterine cavity, i.e. longer than 10 cm in length (clinically similar to a 12-wk pregnant uterus.

Polypectomy and myomectomy, issues include transmural lesions, use of hypotonic media in patients with hyponatremia, use of glycine in patients with liver disease, and use of sorbitol in patients with severe diabetes.

In the following conditions, although hysteroscopy is not contraindicated, it must be done with great care or with special arrangements:

– Extensive intrauterine adhesions: there is increased risk of uterine perforation during inspection or dissection of extensive intrauterine adhesions.

– Stenosed cervix: as in cases following cone biopsy or pelvic irradiation, which may limit of cervical dilatation.

EFFICACY OF HYSTEROSCOPY

Diagnostic hysteroscopy is a simple and safe procedure permitting direct visualization of the uterine cavity on an outpatient basis.

Displaying the hysteroscopic image simultaneously to the physician and the patient helps to explain the diagnosis to the patient, presumably increasing satisfaction and compliance to subsequent treatment.

Diagnostic hysteroscopy has now replaced conventional D&C for the evaluation of the uterine cavity.

Diagnostic hysteroscopy is a reliable tool for the detection of uterine fibroids, endometrial polyps, congenital uterine malformations, synechiae, and complete Asherman's syndrome and provides precise diagnosis of other lesions, previously detected by ultrasound.

Hysteroscopic examination is superior to hysterography in evaluating the endometrial cavity, it has been proven to have superior sensitivity and specificity in evaluating the endometrial cavity, in many practices, diagnostic hysteroscopy is the preferred procedure for the diagnosis of uterine pathology in infertile patients.

Hysteroscopy should be performed especially in patients older than 35 years of age and/or with a history of two or more previous ART trials even in the presence of a normal HSG.

REFERENCES

- Adamson G, Baker V. Subfertility: causes, treatment and outcome. Best Pract Res Clin Obstet Gynaecol. 2003; 17: 169.

- Advincula A, Wang K. Evolving role and current state of robotics in minimally invasive gynecologic surgery. J Minim Invasive Gynecol. 2009; 16: 291.

- American College of Obstetricians and Gynecologists. ACOG technical bulletin: hysteroscopy. Int J. Gynaecol. Obstet. 1994; 45: 175.

- American College of Obstetricians and Gynecologists. Technology assessment in obstetrics and gynecology: hysteroscopy. Obstet Gynecol. 2005; 106: 439.

- American College of Obstetricians and Gynecologists. ACOG practice bulletin: alternatives to hysterectomy in the management of leiomyomas. Obstet Gynecol. 2008; 112.

- American Society for Reproductive Medicine. Optimal evaluation of the infertile female. Fertil Steril. 2006b; 86: S264.

- Ananthanarayan C, Paek W, Rolbin S, et al. Hysteroscopy and anaesthesia. Can J Anaesth. 1996; 43: 56.

- Andreoli M, Servakov M, Meyers P, et al. Laparoscopic surgery during pregnancy. J Am Assoc Gynecol Laparosc. 1999; 6: 229.

- Bacsko G. Uterine surgery by operative hysteroscopy. Eur J Obstet Gynecol Reprod Biol. 1997; 71: 219.

- Baggish K, Karram M. Atlas of pelvic anatomy and gynecologic surgery. Philadelphia, PA: Saunders, Elsevier; 2006.

REFERENCES

- Baggish M, Guedj H, Valle R. Hysteroscopy: visual perspectives of uterine anatomy, physiology and pathology. Philadelphia: Wolters Kluwer Health / Lippincott Williams & Wilkins; 2007.

- Balasch J, Creus M, Fabregues F, et al. Visible and non-visible endometriosis at laparoscopy in fertile and infertile women and in patients with chronic pelvic pain: a prospective study. Hum Reprod. 1996; 11: 387.

- Bettocchi S, Ceci O, Di Venere R, et al. Advanced operative office hysteroscopy without anaesthesia: analysis of 501 cases treated with a 5 Fr. bipolar electrode, Hum Reprod. 2002; 17: 2435.

- Bettocchi S, Ceci O, Nappi L, et al. Operative office hysteroscopy without anesthesia: analysis of 4863 cases performed with mechanical instruments. J Am Assoc Gynecol Laparosc. 2004; 11: 59.

- Bettocchi S, Ceci O, Nappi L, et al. Office hysteroscopic metroplasty: three "diagnostic criteria" to differentiate between septate and bicornuate uteri. J Minim Invasive Gynecol. 2007; 14: 324.

- Bettocchi S, Nappi L, Ceci O, et al., What does "diagnostic hysteroscopy" mean today? The role of the new techniques. Curr Opin Obstet Gynecol. 2003; 15: 303.

- Bettocchi S, Nappi L, Ceci O, et al. Office hysteroscopy. Obstet Gynecol Clin N Am. 2004; 31, 641.

- Bettocchi S, Nappi L, Di Spiezio Sardo A, et al. Effectiveness of hysteroscopy versus transvaginal ultrasound in diagnosing intra-uterine lesions in infertile women. European Obstetrics & Gynaecology. 2008; 3: 12.

- Bettochi S, Selvaggi L. A vaginoscopic approach to reduce the pain of office hysteroscopy. J Am Assoc Gynecol Laparosc. 1997; 4: 255.

REFERENCES

- Boike G, Miller C, Spiritos N, et al. Incisional bowel herniations after operative laparoscopy: a series of nineteen cases and review of the literature. Am J Obstet Gynecol. 1995; 172: 1726.

- Bradley L, Widrich T. Flexible hysteroscopy a state of theart procedure for gynaecologic evaluation. J Am Assoc Gynaecol Laparosc. 1995; 2: 263.

- Bradley L. Complications in hysteroscopy: prevention, treatment and legal risk. Curr Opin Obstet Gynecol. 2002; 14: 409.

- Bradley L. Cutting the risk of hysteroscopic complications. Obg management. 2004; 16: 1.

- Bradley L. Overview of Hysteroscopy. Up-to-date. 2010.

- Bras J. Fluid Overload after Hysteroscopic Polypectomy. Brazilian Journal of Videoendoscopic Surgery. 2010; 3: 90.

- Brill A, Nezhat F, Nezhat C, et al. The incidence of adhesions after prior laparotomy: a laparoscopic appraisal. Obstet Gynecol. 1995; 85: 269.

- Broome J, Vancaillie T. Fluoroscopically guided hysteroscopic division of adhesions in severe Asherman syndrome. Obstet Gynecol. 1999; 93: 1041.

- Brown S, Coddington C, Schnorr J, et al. Evaluation of outpatient hysteroscopy, saline infusion hysterosonography, and hysterosalpingography in infertile women: a prospective randomized study. Fertil Steril. 2000; 74: 1029.

- Brusco G, Arena S, Angelini A. The role of diagnostic hysteroscopy in infertile women. Minerva Gynecol. 2001; 53: 313.

- Bukulmez O, Yarali H, Gurgan T. Total corporal synechiae due to tuberculosis carry a very poor prognosis following hysteroscopic synechialysis. Hum Reprod. 1999; 14: 1960.

REFERENCES

- Campo R, Molinas C, Rombauts L, et al. Prospective multicentre randomized controlled trial to evaluate factors influencing the success rate of office diagnostic hysteroscopy. Hum Reprod. 2005; 20: 258.

- Campo R, Van Belle Y, Rombauts L, et al. Office mini-hysterocopy. Hum Reprod Update. 1999; 5: 73.

- Chaffkin L, Luciano L. Ureteral injuries. In: Corfman R, Diamond W, DeCherney A (eds.). Complications of Laparoscopy and Hysteroscopy. Cambridge, UK: Blackwell; 1993.

- Chew S, Chan C, Ng S, et al. Laparoscopic adhesiolysis for subfertility. Singapore Med J. 1998; 39: 491.

- Chudnoff S, Einstein M, Levie M. Paracervical block efficacy in office hysteroscopic sterilization: a randomized controlled trial. Obstet Gynecol. 2010; 115: 26.

- Chung C, Curry N, Williamson H, et al. Bilateral Fallopian tubal polyps: radiologic and pathologic correlation. Urol Radiol. 1990; 12: 120.

- Cicinelli E, Parisi C, Galantino P, et al. Reliability, feasibility, and safety of minihysterosocpy with a vaginoscopic approach: experience with 6,000 cases. Fertil Steril. 2003; 80: 199.

- Cicinelli E, Pinto V, Tinelli R, et al. Rapid endometrial preparation for hysteroscopic surgery with oral desogestrel plus vaginal raloxifene: a prospective, randomized pilot study. Fertil Steril. 2007; 88: 698.

- Cicinelli E, Resta L, Nicoletti R, et al. Detection of chronic endometritis at fluid hysteroscopy. J Minim Invasive Gynecol. 2005; 12: 514.

- Cicinelli E, Resta L, Nicoletti R, et al. Endometrial micropolyps at fluid hysteroscopy suggest the existence of chronic endometritis. Hum Reprod. 2005; 20: 1386.

REFERENCES

- Cicinelli E. Diagnostic minihysteroscopy with vaginoscopic approach: rationale and advantages. J Minim Invasive Gynecol. 2005; 12: 396.

- Cooper J, Brady R. Intraoperative and early postoperative complications of operative hysteroscopy. Obstet Gynecol Clin N Am. 2000; 27: 347.

- Cooper J, Brady R. Late complications of operative hysteroscopy. Obstet Gynecol Clin N Am. 2000; 27: 367.

- Cooper N, Smith P, Khan K, et al. A systematic review of the effect of the distension medium on pain during outpatient hysteroscopy. Fertil Steril. 2011; 95: 264.

- Corfman R. Indications for hysteroscopy. Obstet Gynecol Clin N Am. 1988; 15: 41.

- Crawford D, Phillips E. Laparoscopic repair and groin hernia surgery. Surg Clin North Am. 1998; 78: 1047.

- Dalal R, Pai H, Palshetkar N, et al. Hysteroscopic metroplasty in women with primary infertility and septate uterus: reproductive performance after surgery. J Reprod Med. 2012; 57: 13.

- De Angelis C, Santoro G, Re M, et al. Office hysteroscopy and compliance: mini-hysteroscopy versus traditional hysteroscopy in a randomized trial. Hum Reprod. 2003b; 18: 2441.

- De Iaco P, Marabini A, Stefanetti M. Acceptability and pain of outpatient hysteroscopy. J Am Assoc Gynecol Laparosc. 2000; 7: 71.

- Dendrinos S, Grigoriou O, Sakkas E, et al. Hysteroscopy in the evaluation of habitual abortions. Eur J Contracept Reprod Health Care. 2008; 13: 198.

- DeSimone C, Ueland F. Gynecologic Laparoscopy. Surgical Clinics of North America. 2008; 88: 66.

REFERENCES

- Di Spiezio S, Mazzon I, Bramante S, et al. Hysteroscopic myomectomy: a comprehensive review of surgical techniques. Hum Reprod Update. 2008; 14: 101.

- Doldi N, Persico P, Di Sebastiono F, et al. Pathologic findings in hysteroscopy before IVF-ET. Gynecol Endocrinol. 2005; 21: 235.

- El-Mazny A, Abou-Salem N, El-Sherbiny W, et al. Outpatient hysteroscopy: a routine investigation before assisted reproductive techniques? Fertil Steril. 2011; 95: 272.

- Emanuel M, Verdel M, Wamsteker K. A prospective comparison of transvaginal ultrasonography and diagnostic hysteroscopy in the evaluation of patients with AUB: clinical implications. Am J Obstet Gynecol. 1995; 172: 547.

- Felemban A, Tan S, Tulandi T. Laparoscopic treatment of polycystic ovaries with insulated needle cautery: a reappraisal. Fertil Steril. 2000; 73: 266.

- Filogônio I, Ávila I, Gouvea P, et al. Accuracy of Hysteroscopic View in the Diagnosis of Intrauterine Pathology: A Brazilian Experience. Journal of Gynecologic Surgery. 2010; 26: 23.

- Floris S, Piras B, Orrù M, et al. Efficacy of intravenous tramadol treatment for reducing pain during office diagnostic hysteroscopy. Fertil Steril. 2007; 87: 147.

- Garbin O, Kutnahorsky R, Göllner J, et al. Vaginoscopic versus conventional approaches to outpatient diagnostic hysteroscopy: a two-centre randomized prospective study. Hum Reprod. 2006; 21: 2996.

- Georgy F, Fetterman H, Chefetz M. Complications of laparoscopy: two cases of perforated urinary bladder. Am J Obstet Gynecol. 1974; 120: 1121.

- Gimpelson R. Hysteroscopic treatment of the patient with intracavitary pathology (myomectomy / polypectomy). Obstet Gynecol Clin N Am. 2000; 27: 327.

REFERENCES

- Giorda G, Scarabelli C, Franceschi S, et al. Feasibility and pain control in outpatient hysteroscopy in postmenopausal women: a randomized trial. Acta Obstet Gynecol Scand. 2000; 79: 593.

- Gomel V, Taylor P. Diagnostic and operative laparoscopy. St. Louis, MO: CV Mosby; 1995.

- Grainger D, Soderstrom R, Schiff S, et al. Ureteral injuries at laparoscopy: insights into diagnosis, management, and prevention. Obstet Gynecol. 1990; 75: 839.

- Grimbizis G, Camus M, Tarlatzis B, et al. Clinical implications of uterine malformations and hysteroscopic treatment results. Hum Reprod. 2001; 7: 161.

- Groenman F, Peters L, Rademaker B, et al. Embolism of air and gas in hysteroscopic procedures: pathophysiology and implication for daily practice. J Minim Invasive Gynecol. 2008; 15: 241.

- Grove J, Shinaman R, Drover D. Noncardiogenic pulmonary edema and venous air embolus as complications of operative hysteroscopy. J Clin Anesth. 2004; 16: 48.

- Grow D, Iromloo K. Oral contraceptives maintain a very thin endometrium before operative hysteroscopy. Fertil Steril. 2006; 85: 204.

- Hamou J, Lewis V. Hysteroscopy and microhysteroscopy. In: Recent advances in obstetrics and gynecology. Longman Group UK Limited; 1991.

- Hasson H, Rotman C, Rana N, et al. Open laparoscopy: 29-year experience. Obstet Gynecol. 2000; 96: 763.

- Hucke J, De Bruyme T, Balan P. Hysteroscopy in infertility diagnosis and treatment including falloscopy. Gynecol Obstet. 2000; 20:.13.

- Hulka J, Reich H. Textbook of laparoscopy. WB Saunders Company; 1998.

REFERENCES

- Hurd W, Amesse L, Gruber J, et al. Visualization of the bladder and epigastric vessels prior to trocar placement in diagnostic and operative laparoscopy. Fertil Steril. 2003; 80: 209.

- Hurd W, Falcone T, Sharp Howard T, et al. Gynecologic Laparoscopy. eMedicine Clinical Procedures. 2009.

- Irvin W, Andersen W, Taylor P, et al. Minimizing the risk of neurologic injury in gynecologic surgery. Obstet Gynecol. 2004; 103: 374.

- Istre O. Managing bleeding, fluid absorption and uterine perforation at hysteroscopy. Best Practice Reseatch Clin Obstet Gynecol. 2009; 23: 619.

- Jansen F, de Kroon C, van Dongen H, et al. Diagnostic hysteroscopy and saline infusion sonography: prediction of intrauterine polyps and myomas. J Minim Invasive Gynecol. 2006; 13: 320.

- Jansen F, Vredevoogd C, van Ulzen K, et al. Complications of hysteroscopy: a prospective, multicenter study. Obstet Gynecol. 2000; 96: 266.

- Kaali S. Establishment of primary port without insertion of a sharp trocar. J Am Assoc Gynecol Laparosc. 1998; 5: 193.

- Kaiser A, Corman M. History of laparoscopy. Surg Oncol Clin N Am. 2001; 10: 482.

- Kandil M, Selim M. Hormonal and sonographic assessment of ovarian reserve before and after laparoscopic ovarian drilling in PCOS. Int J Obstet Gynecol. 2005; 112: 1427.

- Kitajima M. Laparoscopic surgery. Nippon Naika Gakkai Zasshi. 2002; 91: 535.

- Kremer C, Duffy S, Moroney M. Patient satisfaction with outpatient hysteroscopy versus day case hysteroscopy: randomized controlled trial. Br Med J. 2000; 320: 279.

REFERENCES

- Kumar A, Ghadir S, Eskandari N, et al. Infertility. In: Decherney A, Nathan L (eds). Current Diagnosis & Treatment Obstetrics & Gynecology. McGraw-Hill Companies Inc; 2007.

- Kumar S, Awasthi M, Gokhale N. Assessment of Uterine Factor in Infertile Women: hysterosalpingography versus hysteroscopy. MJAFI. 2003; 60: 39.

- Landman J, Kerbl K, Rehman J, et al. Evaluation of a vessel sealing system, bipolar electrosurgery, harmonic scalpel, titanium clips, endoscopic gastrointestinal anastomosis vascular staples & sutures for arterial & venous ligation in a porcine model. J Urol. 2003; 169: 697.

- Lau W, Ho R, Tsang M, et al. Patients acceptance of outpatient hysteroscopy. Gynecol Obstet Invest. 1999; 47: 191.

- Litta P, Bonora M, Pozzan C, et al. Carbon dioxide versus normal saline in outpatient hysteroscopy. Hum Reprod. 2003; 18: 2446.

- Litynski G. Laparoscopy -- the early attempts: spotlighting Georg Kelling and Hans Christian Jacobaeus. JSLS. 1997; 1: 83.

- Loffer F. Endoscopy in high risk patients. In: Martin DC (ed.), Manual of Endoscopy. Santa Fe Springs, CA: American Association of Gynecologic Laparoscopists; 1990.

- Loffer F. Contraindications and complications of hysteroscopy. Obstet Gynecol Clin N Am. 1995; 22: 445.

- Loffer F, Bradley L, Brill A, et al. Hysteroscopic fluid monitoring guidelines. The ad hoc committee on hysteroscopic training guidelines of the American Association of Gynecologic Laparoscopists. J Am Assoc Gynecol Laparosc. 2000; 7: 167.

- Lu P, Liu F, Qi Z. A century of developmental history of laparoscopic surgery. Zhonghua Yi Shi Za Zhi. 2001; 31: 217.

REFERENCES

- Luciano A, Lowney J, Jacobs S. Endoscopic treatment of endometriosis-associated infertility: therapeutic, economic and social benefits. J Reprod Med. 1992; 37: 573.

- Magos A. Hysteroscopic treatment of Asherman's syndrome. Reprod Biomed Online. 2002; 4: 46.

- Magos A. Hysteroscopy and Laparoscopy. In: Dewhurst's Textbook of Obstetrics & Gynaecology, 7th ed., Blacjwell Publishing. 2007.

- Malinowski A, Szpakowski M, Kolasa D, et al. Laparoscopy in pregnancy women. Gynecol Pol. 2002; 73: 247.

- Marana R, Marana E, Catalano G. Current practical application of office endoscopy. Curr Opin Obstet Gynecol. 2001; 13: 383.

- March C. Hysteroscopy. J Reprod Med. 1992; 37: 293.

- Marlow J. Media and delivery systems. Obstet Gynecol Clin N Am. 1995; 22: 409.

- Mettler L, Semm K, Shive K. Endoscopic management of adnexal masses. J Soc Laparoendosc Surg. 1997; 1: 103.

- Molander P, Cacciatore B, Sjoberg J, et al. Laparoscopic management of suspected acute pelvic inflammatory disease. J Am Assoc Gynecol Laparosc. 2007; 7: 107.

- Mollo A, De Franciscis P, Colacurci N, et al. Hysteroscopic resection of the septum improves the pregnancy rate of women with unexplained infertility: a prospective controlled trial. Fertil Steril. 2009; 91: 2628.

- Montz F, Holschneider C, Munro M. Incisional hernia following laparoscopy: a survey of the American Association of Gynecologic Laparoscopists. Obstet Gynecol. 1994; 84: 881.

- Moore S, Green C, Wang F, et al. The role of irrigation in the development of hypothermia during laparoscopic surgery. Am J Obstet Gynecol. 1997; 176: 598.

REFERENCES

- Mouton W, Bessell J, Millard S, et al. A randomized controlled trial assessing the benefit of humidified insufflation gas during laparoscopic surgery. Surg Endosc. 1999; 13: 106.

- Munro M, Brill A, Parker W. Gynecologic Endoscopy, Operative Gynecology. In: Berek & Novak's Gynecology. Lippincott Williams & Wilkins; 2007.

- Nagele F, Bournas N, O'Connor H, et al. Comparison of CO2 and normal saline for uterine distension in outpatint hysteroscopy. Fertil Steril. 1996; 65: 305.

- Nagele F, Lockwood G, Magos A. Randomized placebo controlled trial of mefenamic acid for premedication at outpatient hysteroscopy: a pilot study. Br J Obstet Gynaecol. 1997; 104, 842.

- Nagele F, O'Connor H, Davies A, et al. Two thousand five hundred outpatient diagnostic hysteroscopies. Obstet Gynecol. 1996; 88: 87.

- Nawroth F, Foth D, Schmidt T. Minihysteroscopy as a routine diagnostic procedure in women with primary infertility. J Am Assoc Gynecol Laparosc. 2003; 10: 396.

- Nezhat C, Nezhat C, Nezhat F, et al. Principles of Laparoscopy. In: Nezhat's Operative Gynecologic Laparoscopy and Hysteroscopy. Cambridge University Press; 2008.

- Nezhat C, Nezhat F, Nezhat C. Operative laparoscopy (minimally invasive surgery): state of the art. J. Gynecol Surg. 1992; 8: 111.

- Nezhat C, Nezhat F, Nezhat C. Complications of laparoscopic surgery. In: Asch R, Studd J (eds.). Progress in Reproductive Medicine. The Parthonen Pub. Group; 1995.

- Nezhat C, Siegler A, Nezhat F, et al. Equipment. In: Operative Gynecologic Laparoscopy: Principles and Techniques; 2000.

REFERENCES

- Nezhat F, Brill A, Nezhat C, et al. Laparoscopic appraisal of the anatomic relationship of the umbilicus to the aortic bifurcation. J Am Assoc Gynecol Laparosc. 1998; 5: 135.

- Nezhat F, Tazuke S, Nezhat C, et al. Laparoscopy during pregnancy: A literature review. J Soc Laparoendosc Surg. 1997; 1: 17.

- Ngai S, Chan Y, Ho P. The use of misoprostol prior to hysteroscopy in postmenopausal women. Hum Reprod. 2001; 16: 1486.

- Ocampo J, Nutis M, Nezhat C, et al. Equipment. In: Nezhat's Operative Gynecologic Laparoscopy and Hysteroscop. Cambridge University Press; 2008.

- O'Donovan P, McGurgan P. Microlaparoscopy. Semin laparosc Surg. 1999; 6: 51.

- Ostrzenski A, Radolmski B, Ostrzenski K. A review of laparoscopic uretal injury in pelvic surgery. Obstet Gynecol Surv. 2003; 58: 794.

- Ozgur K, Isikoglu M, Donmez L, et al. Is hysteroscopic correction of an incomp.lete uterine septum justified prior to IVF? Reprod Biomed Online. 2007; 14: 335.

- Pabuccu R, Atay V, Orhon E, et al. Hysteroscopic treatment of intrauterine adhesions is safe and effective in the restoration of normal menstruation and fertility. Fertil Steril. 1997; 68: 1141.

- Palmer R. Safety in laparoscopy. J Reprod Med. 1974; 13: 1.

- Paraiso M, Walters M. Laparoscopic pelvic reconstructive surgery. Clin Obstet Gynecol. 2000; 43: 594.

- Paschopoulos M, Kaponis A, Makrydimas G, et al. Selecting distending medium for out-patient hysteroscopy. Does it really matter? Hum Reprod. 2004; 19: 2619.

REFERENCES

- Pellicano M, Guida M, Zullo F, et al. Carbon dioxide versus normal saline as a uterine distention medium for diagnostic vaginoscopic hysteroscopy in infertile patients: a prospective, randomized, multicenter study. Fertil Steril. 2003; 79: 418.

- Perez-Medina T, Bajo-Arenas J, Martinez-Cortes L, et al. Six thousand office diagnostic-operative hysteroscopies. Int J Gynecol Obstet. 2000; 71: 33.

- Peterson H, Hulka J, Phillips J. American Association of Gynecologic Laparoscopists' 1988 membership survey on operative laparoscopy. J Reprod Med. 1990; 35: 587.

- Phillips J. Laparoscopy. Baltimore: Williams & Wilkins; 1997.

- Preutthipan S, Linasmita V. Reproductive outcome following hysteroscopic lysis of intrauterine adhesions: a result of 65 cases at Ramathibodi Hospital. J Med Assoc Thai. 2000; 83: 42.

- Promecene P. Laparoscopy in gynecologic emergencies. Semin Laparosc Sug. 2002; 9: 64.

- Propst A, Liberman R, Harlow B, et al. Complications of hysteroscopic surgery: predicting patients at risk. Obstet Gynecol. 2000; 96: 517.

- Raiga J, Canis M, Le Bouedec G, et al. Laparoscopic management of adnexal abscesses: consequences for fertility. Fertil Steril. 1996; 66: 712.

- Ray G. The effectiveness of laparoscopic excision of endometriosis. Curr Opin Obstet Gynecol. 2004; 16: 299.

- Readman E, Maher P. Pain relief and outpatient hysteroscopy: a literature review. J Am Assoc Gynecol Laparosc. 2004; 11: 315.

- Revel A, Shushan A. Investigation of infertile: hysteroscopy with endometrial biopsy is the gold standard investigation for abnormal uterine bleeding. Human Reprod. 2002; 17: 1947.

REFERENCES

- Risquez F, Confino E. Transcervical tubal cannulation, past, present and future. Fertil Steril. 1993; 60: 211.

- Rojansky N, Shushan A, Fatum M. Laparoscopy versus laparotomy in pregnancy: a comparative study. J Am Assoc Gynecol Laparosc. 2002; 9: 108.

- Ross J. Numerous indications for office flexible minihysteroscopy. J Am Assoc Gynecol Laparosc. 2000; 7: 221.

- Salat-Baroux J, Hamou J, Maillard G, et al. Complications from microhysteroscopy. In: Siegler A, Lindemann J (eds). Hysteroscopy. Philadelphia, JB: Lippincott; 1984.

- Sanfilippo J, Roberts L. Laparoscopic Surgery in Danforth's Obstetrics and Gynecology. Lippincott Williams & Wilkins; 2008.

- Schaller G, Kuenkel M, Manegold B. The optical "Veress-needle"- initial puncture with a minioptic. Endosc Surg Allied Technol. 1995; 3: 55.

- Schenk L, Coddington C. Laparoscopy and hysteroscopy. Obstet Gynecol Clin N Am. 1999; 26: 1.

- Schorge J, Schaffer J, Halvorson L, et al. Williams Gynecology. New York: McGraw-Hill Medical; 2008.

- Seidman, Berker B, Nezhat C. Management of tubo-ovarian abcesses, Management of adnexal masses. In: Nezhat's Operative Gynecologic Laparoscopy and Hysteroscopy. Cambridge University Press; 2008.

- Shankar M, Davidson A, Taub N, et al. Randomised comparison of distension media for outpatient hysteroscopy. BJOG. 2004; 111: 57.

- Sharma M, Taylor A, Di Spiezio S, et al. Outpatient hysteroscopy: traditional versus the "no-touch" technique. BJOG. 2005; 112: 963.

REFERENCES

- Shokeir T, Shalan H, El-Shafei M. Significance of endometrial polyps detected hysteroscopically in eumenorrheic infertile women. J Obstet Gynaecol Res. 2004: 30: 84.

- Shveiky D, Rojansky N, Revel A, et al. Complications of hysteroscopic surgery: "Beyond the learning curve". J Minim Invasive Gynecol. 2007; 14: 218.

- Siegler J. Office hysteroscopy. Obstet Gynecol Clin N Am. 1995; 22: 457.

- Soderstrom R. Electrosurgical injuries during laparoscopy: prevention and management. Curr Opin Obstet Gynecol. 1994; 6: 248.

- Speroff L, Glass R, Kase N. Female infertility. In: Speroff L, Glass R, Kase N (eds). Clinical Gynecologic Endocrinology and Infertility. Philadelphia, PA: Lippincott Williams & Wilkins; 2005.

- Spiewankiewicz B, Stelmachow J, Sawicki W, et al. The effectiveness of hysteroscopic polypectomy in cases of female infertility. Clin Exp Obstet Gynecol. 2003; 30: 23.

- Stamatellos I, Apostolides A, Stamatopoulos P, et al. Pregnancy rates after hysteroscopic polypectomy depending on the size or number of the polyps. Arch Gynecol Obstet. 2008; 277: 395.

- Stany M, Farley J. Complications of gynecologic surgery. Surg Clin N Am. 2008; 88: 343.

- Swanström L. Natural orifice transluminal endoscopic surgery. Endoscopy. 2009; 41: 82.

- Tam W, Lau W, Cheung L, et al. Intrauterine adhesions after conservative and surgical management of spontaneous abortion. J Am Assoc Gynecol Laparosc. 2002; 9: 182.

REFERENCES

- Taşkın E, Berker B, Ozmen B, et al. Comparison of hysterosalpingography and hysteroscopy in the evaluation of the uterine cavity in patients undergoing assisted reproductive techniques. Fertil Steril. 2011; 96: 349.

- Taskin O, Sadik S, Onoglu A, et al. Role of endometrial suppression on the frequency of intrauterine adhesions after resectoscopic surgery. J Am Assoc Gynecol Laparosc. 2000; 3: 351.

- Taylor E, Gomel V. The uterus and fertility. Fertil Steril. 2008; 89: 1.

- Teng F, Muzsnai D, Perez R, et al. A comparative study of laparoscopy and colpotomy for the removal of ovarian dermoid cysts. Obstet Gynecol. 1996; 87: 1009.

- Tham M, Copperman A. Surgical management of polycystic ovarian syndrome, management of adnexal masses. In: Nezhat's Operative Gynecologic Laparoscopy and Hysteroscopy. Cambridge University Press; 2008.

- Thomson A, Abbott J, Kingston A, et al. Fluoroscopically guided synechiolysis for patients with Asherman's syndrome: menstrual and fertility outcomes. Fertil Steril. 2007; 87: 405.

- Thurmond A, Jones M, Cohen D, et al. Procedures for diagnosis and treatment of infertility. In: Gynecologic, Obstetric and Breast Radiology. Cambridge: Blackwell Science; 1996.

- Unfried G, Wieser F, Albrecht A, et al. Flexible versus rigid endoscopes for outpatient hysteroscopy: a prospective randomized clinical trial. Hum Reprod. 2001; 16: 168.

- Valle R. A Manual of Clinical Hysteroscopy. New York: Parthenon Publishing; 1998.

- Van Der Pas H, Vancaille T. Manual of hysteroscopy. Amsterdam; 1990.

REFERENCES

- Van Dongen H, de Kroon C, Jacobi C, et al. Diagnostic hysteroscopy in abnormal uterine bleeding: a systematic review and meta-analysis. BJOG. 2007; 114: 664.

- Vecchio R, MacFayden B, Palazzo F. History of laparoscopic surgery. Panminerva Med. 2000; 42: 87.

- Vercellini P, Zaina B, Yaylayan L, et al. Hysteroscopic myomectomy: long-term effects on menstrual pattern and fertility. Obstet Gynecol. 1999; 94: 341.

- Vilos G, Abu-Rafea B. New developments in ambulatory hysteroscopic surgery. Best Pract Res Clin Obstet Gynaecol. 2005; 19: 727.

- Viswanathan M, Hartmann K, McKoy N, et al. Management of uterine fibroids: an update of the evidence. Evidence Report/Technology Assessment. 2007; 154: 1.

- Wieser F, Kurz C, Wenzl R, et al. Atraumatic cervical passage at outpatient hysteroscopy. Fertil Steril. 1998; 69: 549.

- Wieser F, Tempfer C, Kurz C, et al. Hysteroscopy in 2001: a comprehensive review. Acta Obstet Gynecol Scand. 2001; 80: 773.

- Wong A, Wong K, Tang L. Stepwise pain score analysis of the effect of local lignocaine on outpatient hysteroscopy: a randomized, double-blind, placebo-controlled trial. Fertil Steril. 2000; 73: 1234.

- Yang J, Vollenhoven B. Pain control in outpatient hysteroscopy. Obstet Gynecol Surv. 2002; 37: 693.

www.ingramcontent.com/pod-product-compliance
Lightning Source LLC
Chambersburg PA
CBHW070159230526
45471CB00002B/736